TIGER, TRUE TO FORM

Written by ELLEN S. KANG

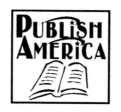

PublishAmerica
Baltimore

ISBN: 1-4241-1017-3
PUBLISHED BY PUBLISHAMERICA, LLLP
www.publishamerica.com
Baltimore

Printed in the United States of America

Dedication

Dedicated to the memories of the good souls who contributed to Andrew Ho Kang's life and success, both in Korea and the United States of America. They are figured in this work, citing their special contributions without which the distinctions of Tiger might not have blossomed.

TABLE OF CONTENTS

CHAPTER 1   JUNE 25, 1950   7
CHAPTER 2   FATHER'S DILEMMA   13
CHAPTER 3   EVASION AND CAPTURE   22
CHAPTER 4   INCARCERATION AND FREEDOM   34
CHAPTER 5   MOTHER, OH, MOTHER!   40
CHAPTER 6   EVACUATION TO THE SOUTH   51
CHAPTER 7   RETURN, CONVERSION AND A
             BREAK   58
CHAPTER 8   TIGER GOES WEST   68
CHAPTER 9   WOFFORD COLLEGE AND
             SPARTANBURG, S.C.   93
CHAPTER 10   HARVARD AND THE GIRL FROM
             HAWAII   108
CHAPTER 11   RUDE ENCOUNTER WITH ARTHRITIS   116
CHAPTER 12   FAMILY AND CAREER SHAPING   125
CHAPTER 13   BACK TO THE SOUTH   137
CHAPTER 14   RETURN TO ASIA AND BACK   145
CHAPTER 15   CHAIRMAN OF MEDICINE   151
CHAPTER 16   BACK TO FULL-TIME RESEARCH   155
CHAPTER 17   CREDITS   163

CHAPTER 1: JUNE 25, 1950

Reaching for his Chinese dictionary, Tiger heard the thud, thud again. Surely, it must be a thunderstorm announcing the beginning of the monsoons, he thought to himself. It was already the 25th of June and rain would be expected to keep the rice crops and farmers happy. But the sounds were not randomly intermittent, as might be expected with a thunderstorm. Instead, their constancy and unnatural rhythmicity suggested something man-made.

Perhaps, the government is blasting a new road beyond Grandfather's place at Ui-dong, maybe even moving north of Seoul, he thought. At least, that might make it easier to hike up the mountain, instead of fighting the brush all the way to the base of the mighty rock even before climbing up to the cliff, he continued in thought. He could hardly wait to pick up the challenge of climbing the mountain again with his imagined vision of a cleared path!

Returning to the task at hand, Tiger flipped the pages of the dictionary until he found the calligraphic figure matching the one in the booklet he was reading for the special after school lessons he had been taking in Chinese. Because of the influence of China on various Asian countries and the fact that many Chinese ideographs were adopted by both the Koreans and Japanese, Father had engaged a tutor of Chinese for his Number One Son to extend his education beyond what would be learned in school.

Tiger was a tenth grader at Kyonggi High School for Boys, the most prestigious school for boys in Seoul, where he was an exceptional student. He had been born during the Japanese occupation of Korea and consequently was taught to read and speak Japanese during his entire elementary school education. Invariably though, like other Korean school children, he reverted to Korean at home and amongst his friends. With the liberation of Korea at the end of World War II, Japanese was no longer compulsory for the students of South Korea. Thereafter, English was the language to learn and Tiger had been studying English for the last four years in school. He had also been studying German, so all together, the net time invested toward the acquisition of several language skills was quite substantial for the young man, or for that matter, for anyone of whatever age.

All the while, he continued to excel at school, frequently exceeding assignments because of personal interests that led him to delve into his Father's large collection of classical and historical Korean, Japanese, Chinese, German and English books in their home library. Classes had resumed for the year at the beginning of April and, as might be anticipated, he had excelled on the recent spring examinations.

As the morning passed, the thudding sounds were no longer distant. In fact, several times Tiger felt the floor on which he sat before the low table he was using as a desk vibrate, as though transmitting an earth driven force.

Force, he thought, something like an explosion must be occurring either above or beneath the ground at a close-enough distance to emit such a vibration.

Apprehensive, he got off the floor and walked out of the room, looking for his parents to see if either of them had felt the same and might have an explanation.

"Omoni (Mother), what is that sound I hear and just now felt as a vibration?"

"I don't know, Tiger," she responded, "but Father has been outside to see if it could be the weather or a blasting project nearby. Our neighbor, the surgeon Dr. Kim, has also heard these sounds, and both he and Father have been checking around to find out the basis for the noise and shaking of the ground and buildings."

Shortly thereafter, Tiger's Father returned from his latest exploration outside. He was ashen in color and uttered some words to his wife in a low, ominous tone.

Mother nodded her head with a worried look on her face and then summarily went about gathering everyone living in the doctor's house into the main room.

Before long everyone was seated on the matted floor wondering what was going on in view of the sounds each had also heard. They were facing the doctor who was already seated apart from the family and household helpers, appearing troubled and concerned.

"The sounds we've been hearing are those of gunfire and explosives. The Communists from the North are blasting us, attacking our troops at the border. They have apparently crossed the 38th parallel and are headed toward Seoul right now, even as we are talking!" he said with a look of deep consternation and alarm, all mixed together.

He continued, "We must all remain indoors, off the streets, preferably in this room, which is structurally the strongest room in the house."

"To-oma" (a distant relative of theirs, who was living and

helping the family) "and the rest of our helpers will have to assist Mother to obtain as much non-perishable food items as we can acquire. You must also collect and store drinking water in case of a long siege, remove flammable items away from the house, as well as rearrange our sleeping quarters, keeping as many as possible near this central room. There will be other precautions that must be taken and each of you must help Mother to accomplish them," he continued.

"In the meantime, we must keep our eyes peeled and let everyone know where we are at all times."

"As for me, I must round up the cadre of anti-Communists we have organized to keep watch over our neighborhood against possible infiltrators and saboteurs, so I shall be away."

A few moments of quiet followed as the adults tried to grasp the suddenness with which their fortune of peaceful living had, for all intents and purposes, vanished. All the fears aroused by the unnerving disagreement prior to the settlement of the division of Korea into a Communist North and a free South were rekindled, sparked by visions of conflict as announced by the sounds of the advancing war. Even the children were quiet, sensing that all was not well.

Before long, Tiger's Father was gone.

Mother dispatched two of her household workers and To-oma to fetch staples from various local shops. She cautioned each to keep to the building walls and shadows, away from the streets and open spaces, during the execution of their tasks as she sent them off with monies sufficient for their purchases.

Then she reorganized the storage of various items and reassigned sleeping areas for the family and workers, clustering everyone in or close to the main room located in the center of the house. Water was collected and stored in containers before placement at several sites around the main room. Large cans of kerosene used to light their stove were relegated to the out-house area, away from contact with the structural components of the large house in which the family, relatives and workers of Dr. Kun Ha Kang resided in the up-scale sector of Iksun-dong in Seoul, Korea.

These disruptions of their usual Sunday activities interfered with Tiger's ability to study any further. Instead, he pitched right in with the busy activities going on in the house, preparing for war.

After a generation under the yoke of the Japanese, the citizens of the southern half of the old nation of Choson or Korea had desperately tried to find their way toward freedom.

In 1947, the United Nations Temporary Commission on Korea supervised the transition of the southern half to a democratic form of government, something the people of Korea had never before experienced. A year later, free, nationwide elections were held and on August 15, 1948, the Commission officially established the Republic of Korea, as the only legitimate Korean government recognized by the United Nations. Until now, democracy had only gained a tenuous foothold and the economy was woefully behind.

Shortly thereafter, the U.S. had withdrawn its armed forces, leaving only a remnant to assist the Koreans to train their own men as a hedge against any possibility that the North might invade by crossing the 38th parallel in a move to take over the southern Republic of Korea. This left insufficient time for the struggling new democracy to muster the personnel, let alone the resources, to establish a reasonable force, in either number of men, level of training or the military arms and means to wage even a defensive stance. Consequently, the country's military was both totally unprepared and ill equipped to withstand any sort of an attack in the summer of 1950.

The sounds of distant explosions continued—now in bursts, then intermittently, but constant—never ending. Towards evening after spending the day accomplishing the many necessary tasks, the family sat apprehensively and quietly in the relative dark of the gathering dusk awaiting Father's return.

Earlier, they had been warned to refrain from the use of fire or of lighting any room after dark without blocking the windows with the wooden shutters for fear of attracting the enemy's attention and fire. Dinner had been prepared during the light of day and now, all was ready except for the return of the head of the household, Dr. Kun Ha Kang, an internist whose clinic was located next to the house. There had been a few patients at the clinic, even on this Sunday, the 25th of June in 1950.

Dr. Kang finally arrived and life resumed in a somewhat stilted, restrained manner in the dining area against the backdrop of the sounds of distant warfare. He spoke quietly and with obvious resignation to the uncertainty that lay ahead for each of them. He advised his children to obey their Mother and for Tiger to be the grown-up, responsible Son that he knew he was. Otherwise, he mumbled to his wife who nodded off and on throughout the meal.

Later, there was a bit of welcomed levity and mirth as everyone groped around in the dark to find his way about as a result of the rearrangements that had been agreed upon earlier. How it was that any of them could have fallen asleep might be difficult to imagine. Perhaps it was the rhythmicity of the thudding, or the warmth arising from the knowledge that other members of the family were close by, but sleep finally did come to each of them, even to Dr. Kang.

CHAPTER 2: FATHER'S DILEMNA

On each succeeding day, the sounds of war increased in intensity, heralding the movement of the line of battle ever further southward from the 38th parallel, toward the city of Seoul, the capital of South Korea.

Just three days later on June 28th, street to street fighting was occurring close to the Iksun-dong area, where the Kangs lived.

Everyone huddled and cowered in the main room. Rifle shots and machine gun rat-atat-atats blasted outside in the streets. Several houses around the district were burning, filling the air with acrid odors of burning structural materials mingled with the smell of gunpowder. Now and then horrifying shrieks and rude shouts could be heard that sent curdling shivers and shakes through Tiger's body.

Despite his own anxiety, he would from time to time wrap his arm around his younger brother, Pyo, and his youngest sisters, Bok Im and Kyung Im, to comfort them and quiet their shivering.

"Don't worry, Father is here and will take care of us," he reassured them.

After several hours, the sounds gradually moved away, headed further south before new ones of motor vehicles, trucks and motorcycles replaced those of the receding gunfire.

The city of Seoul fell to the Communists on the 28th of June.

Distant gunfire interrupted the muted sounds of a city under strict Communist Military rule just three days after the Communist forces had crossed the 38th parallel.

Soon there were edicts blaring out of loud speakers perched on vehicles crawling throughout the streets of Seoul imposing Martial Law and issuing a list of commands including a warning for all citizens to relinquish any fire arms, to expose all military personnel, to refrain from street activities, and for all essential personnel (firemen, policemen, doctors and other hospital personnel) to continue to show up for work and to proceed with their activities, and so forth.

Unlike Dr. Kim, the surgeon residing two houses away, who continued to travel daily to Seoul National University Hospital to work, soon caring for injured Communist soldiers, Dr. Kang simply went next door to his own clinic adjoining his home.

Surprisingly, many patients with acute symptoms related to the stress of the war, were already there. His usual staff had been whittled down to the pharmacist and one nurse, who appeared at work to help the doctor. Whether the others had left the city, moving south to escape the Communists, or had been injured, was not clear to anyone. Nevertheless, Dr. Kang proceeded to work and was kept busy nearly all day except for a break for lunch, which was dutifully delivered by To-oma.

This routine was also followed the next day and the mood at home was somewhat more relaxed. Could it be that all the Communists were interested in was to unite the country, not to impose terror and radical change, wondered the doctor's wife, hoping above all odds?

Early on the third day after the fall of Seoul, before breakfast was over, there was a sudden loud banging at the front door frightening everyone.

To-oma raced to the door to open it. She was rudely brushed aside by several charging, armed North Korean soldiers, who barged in demanding everyone to hold still and to point out the man they were looking for, Kang Kun Ha.

The leader pointed his finger at Tiger's Father, who had risen from his seat, and asked menacingly, "Are you Kang Kun Ha?"

As soon as the doctor had acknowledged that he was, one of the men grabbed the doctor's arms, twisted them backward, and tied both of his hands together in the back with a rope, as the doctor's wife rushed forth in protest.

"What are you doing? Why are you doing this? What has he done? Tell me, why you are doing this?" cried his wife with anxious shouts, tugging at the rope with which his hands were bound in a desperate act to unleash him from the tether.

Alarmed, the younger children were crying out loudly in fright for their Father and their Mother. The older children gasped in horror, moving out of the way of the fracas towards the sidewall. To-oma reached for the youngsters, holding the two youngest daughters of the good doctor closely and firmly against her warm body with both of her arms, biting her lower lip in fright as much as in anger at this terrorizing invasion.

The soldiers rudely pushed the doctor's wife aside without answering her pleading questions. Then, they forcibly dragged the doctor by his shirt collar out of the house towards a waiting military vehicle without so much as an explanation to anyone, not even to the doctor himself.

"Where are you taking him? Why don't you take me, too!" pleaded his wife rushing out behind the captors who were prodding her husband with the butts of their rifles toward the military vehicle parked on the street before their home.

Just before they reached the vehicle, the doctor resisted their further prodding, turned around to face his wife and spoke gently to her, asking her to take care of the family during his absence. "I shall return as soon as this mistake is cleared up," he said to reassure her, as well as himself, perhaps.

"Shut up, you bastard!" the leader shouted as he punched the doctor's back and rudely shoved him into the back seat.

"We don't want you, woman, we're after your husband! Now get back off the street, or you shall be charged criminally for interfering with us!" the leader shouted at the doctor's wife pushing her backward and knocking her onto the ground, before stepping into the vehicle himself. He slammed the vehicle door shut. "Let's go!" he barked.

With the engine roaring loudly, they drove off with Dr. Kang in the back, sandwiched between two armed, hostile looking Communist soldiers—the last view Mrs. Kang was to have of her husband.

Mrs. Kang picked herself off the ground and called for her husband by name as she watched them speed off ahead. Slowly and tearfully, she turned toward the gate before the house. Her heart was pounding wildly and she had a deep sense of dread that she might not see her husband again.

Once in the house, Mrs. Kang tried to calm the children, who were wailing and calling for their Father. The household help rushed around, holding one child or another, trying to reassure them that their Father would return forthwith, but without much confidence based on the look on Mrs. Kang's face.

Wiping her own tears with her handkerchief, Mrs. Kang sighed deeply, acknowledging the coming to fruition of the fear that she and her husband had shared in whispers upon the outbreak of the war.

Once the children were quieted down, she quietly asked To-oma to supervise and watch over the family in her stead. She had some important matters to attend to and would have to leave the house for a while. She had to seek the assistance of her brother, who lived close by, she told To-oma.

As she walked cautiously towards her brother's home, keeping along the walls and fences of the houses lining the streets, Mrs. Kang could not help but consider the underlying series of events that culminated in the sudden arrest of her husband.

He had been extremely concerned about the international political negotiations regarding the fate of Korea toward the end of the Second World War. Whereas prior to the end of World War II, Allied intensions to declare independence for Korea upon capitulation of the Japanese had been made initially at Cairo and later confirmed at Potsdam, the behavior of the USSR near the end of the war had been deceitful, altering the preset plan for Korea.

With selfish designs, just days after the Russians had been asked by the Japanese to intervene in seeking a truce with the Allies following the atomic bombing of Hiroshima and Nagasaki, the USSR declared war on Japan. The Russians subsequently sent troops down the peninsula of Korea, reaching the 38th parallel before Japan would finally agree to an unconditional surrender instead of a negotiated settlement, which Japan had asked the Russians to promote.

Russia wanted a foothold on the peninsula of Korea and a seaport on the Pacific that would not become ice-locked during the winter months. Their only Pacific port, Vladivostok, was frequently unusable during the icy months. By declaring war on Japan without having to fire a shot and advancing down the peninsula of Korea, Russia was assured of access to the several port cities of Korea on the Pacific Ocean during the winter months. Thus it was that Korea, now freed from Japan's colonization, was split in two at the 38th parallel, the furthest south the Russians had reached at the time of Japan's unconditional surrender.

There followed a series of messy international negotiations led by the U.S. seeking to allow those in the South to begin to initiate their own government. By 1948, South Korea was declared independent under the auspices of the United Nations Charter.

All the while, the Russians forged ahead to transform the territory above the 38th parallel into a Communist State. The UN decree regarding the Republic of Korea was declared illegal by the Soviets. Instead, the Soviets established formal diplomatic recognition of North Korea alone, which had adopted the farcical eponym, the Democratic People's Republic of Korea or the DPRK.

Following the establishment of the DPRK, North Korea had regularly sent infiltrators across the border to serve as saboteurs, insurgents, and spies, anticipating the coming of a border breach in the not too distant future.

Now, fully armed and trained by the Soviets, the Democratic People's Republic of Korea had sent its militant forces across the 38th parallel, supposedly to unite the country once again, but to ensure its total conversion to a single Communist State.

Her husband was born and raised in Iwon located well above the 38th parallel, along the east coast of the peninsula of Korea. His father was a prosperous landowner, whose property was farmed by many tenant farmers. As the firstborn son of the wealthy farmer, and as Korea was under Japanese occupation, he had been sent to Japan for his education.

She herself, the only daughter of the literary genius and patriot, Choi Nam Sun whose pen name was Yukdang, had also been educated in Japan. She had met the student from Iwon at a gathering of some Koreans studying in Tokyo. Upon completion of her studies, she had returned home to Seoul.

Kun Ha had elected to study medicine, but instead of staying in Japan had returned to Seoul to study at Keijo Imperial University, now renamed Seoul National University.

Of course, she was delighted to learn of Kun Ha's return to Korea and it was not unexpected that she would marry him shortly thereafter.

Three years before the end of World War II, her husband's father had died after a fatal stroke in the northern city of Iwon. Instead of returning to Iwon to supervise the land which he subsequently inherited, her husband had allowed his relatives and the tenant farmers to continue to farm the land, just as his Father had. He received shares of the crops in payment from the tenants of the land and traveled back and forth whenever necessary to oversee family related and financial matters.

After the war and the division of Korea, the Communists confiscated his property and either killed or conscripted many of his relatives and tenant farmers. Several had escaped to the South with terrible stories to tell of the cruelty, injustice, and terror inflicted upon them in Iwon and elsewhere in North Korea. Furthermore, Communist infiltrators were also being sent to the South to sabotage and disrupt the transition of South Korea towards a democracy.

It was during this time that Dr. Kun Ha Kang was motivated to work with the local authorities to organize and supervise neighborhood groups to keep surveillance against such Communist intruders. He had become one of several leaders in these campaigns in Seoul.

Once the invasion had begun, both the doctor and his wife became acutely aware of the possibility that he and others engaged in such activities would likely be singled out for capture by Communist sympathizers. Following the fall of Seoul, they lived with bated breath for the passing of each day in safety and without incarceration.

And, here it was, the worst of their nightmares had just come to pass! There was no way to have evacuated to the south with the speedy progression of the war and the unexpected collapse of their military. Besides, considering the size and circumstances of their extended family, how could they have left under the hail of mortar raining down everywhere!

She made her way carefully to the home of her younger brother, a pediatrician, Dr. Han Woong Choi, who lived with his wife and family, not too far away from Iksun-dong.

She knocked and entered the house. Her agitated and frightened look had gotten her brother's undivided attention. She began to relate the morning's unbelievable occurrence interrupted only by the need to blow her nose, which ran along with her eyes as she cried throughout her telling of the stark brutality of the morning's episode that spelled disaster.

Han Woong knew of his brother-in-law's community activities and realized immediately the odds against which they had to work. Consoling her as best as he could, he consulted his wife and then returned to his older sister's dilemma

Together, they decided to risk traveling to the Police Station of Central Seoul, which had been taken over as a command post for the Communist Military. Traveling by foot, they kept to the shadows of the buildings, away from the open lanes.

The streets were virtually deserted except for North Korean soldiers traveling in pairs with rifles ready who were stalking the streets, looking for suspicious activities. Several North Korean soldiers could be seen here and there questioning men who held their arms up high in great fright.

Finally, they reached the Police Station, which was staffed by North Korean soldiers, as all civilian policemen had fled southward or had been held for indoctrination to the Communist ideals.

Rudely, the North Korean soldiers asked the couple what their business was.

"My name is Choi Han Woong. I am a physician. This lady is my sister. We are looking for Dr. Kun Ha Kang, my brother-in-law and this lady's husband. He is a practicing doctor with many patients dependent on his care. He was illegally taken from his home at Iksun-dong by soldiers this morning."

"We want to know where he is, what the charge is, and we wish to restore him back to our family," said Dr. Han Woong Choi in a calm voice.

"And, what if I tell you that he is a prisoner of the Democratic People's Republic of Korea for counter-revolutionary activities and that he will not be released to anyone at all!" replied the stern-looking commander behind the desk.

"Now, get out of here, the both of you, or we'll have two more prisoners to cope with," he snapped harshly. Whereupon two soldiers dragged Dr. Choi and Mrs. Kang by their collars, leading them out of the hall and rudely shoving them out of the door.

"Get out, go home and stay there, or else!" they warned.

Dr. Choi took Mrs. Kang by the arm. "We're not going to be able to do anything for now. Let us return home and wait. It could be that he might be released after a few days," her brother said, not believing that they would ever see him again, alive or dead.

Carefully, they made their way back to Mrs. Kang's home.

Dr. Choi's appearance at the house brought great comfort to the children who knew him and loved him as their closest relative, like a surrogate father. Besides, Dr. Choi was the father of their immediate cousins with whom they had many social and personal interactions almost on a daily basis.

He spoke reassuring words to each, predicting the return of their Father, unharmed and in good health. He promised to be there for each of them as necessary and then he left to join his own family down the street off Iksun-dong.

CHAPTER 3: EVASION AND CAPTURE

With each passing day, hope of Father's return grew dimmer and dimmer. Attempts to gather information were unsuccessful as were efforts to extend packaged goods for the doctor's needs. These were summarily opened and either eaten or stolen for the various Communists' personal use. Several times they openly draped the articles of clothing against their own bodies and gloated over the edible goods that were sent before shoving the deliverer out through the door, rudely, and without information as to the current whereabouts of Dr. Kang.

Days later one morning, loud orders were blasted out by bullhorn from a military vehicle driving slowly down the various streets of the district where the Kangs lived. All men fourteen years of age and over were ordered to appear at a neighborhood hall that very day.

Tiger's Mother and her good friend, Mrs. Kim, the wife of the surgeon two houses away, consulted with each other. Their sons were classmates and both were over fourteen years of age.

Suspecting this was to identify all possible eligible males for forced consignment into their military or slave work corps, they agreed the boys should report together, stick together, and to use their cunning to escape together using all their wiles and instinctual smarts.

With that, each consulted with her own son, made him promise to stick with the other boy, to keep alert for indications as to whether they would be kept captive, and if so, to seek the best way to escape without arousing suspicion. They had to escape and to return home safely, no two ways about that, they were told and duly forewarned. Upon their return, they were to proceed to Mrs. Kim's home to remain hidden under her orders. Mrs. Kim would keep in touch with Tiger's Mother and both would provide for Tiger's and Myung Ho's needs, they promised.

Somewhat excited about the prospect of an adventure not experienced before, Tiger nodded his head with only a bit of apprehension. His Father had still not returned, but Tiger naively had not abandoned any hope that he would suddenly reappear one day, and soon he believed this would be the case.

After lunch, Mrs. Kang composed Tiger, advising him again about the dangers they might face. When Myung Ho Kim, the surgeon's son, appeared, she reinforced what they had been told and bid both a safe return, promising to keep a close watch for them.

The boys reached the place designated for them to report.

They were almost inappropriately glad to see others of their friends who had also appeared with their elder brothers and fathers. There was a solemnity in the faces of each of the older men however, that restrained them from social interactions, which usually followed such encounters.

One of the soldiers with a bull horn moved them along to form several lines in front of tables behind which sat other solders with sheets of paper. Everyone was asked his name, home address, date of birth, occupation, and whether he had a short list of diseases or handicaps.

Afterwards, each one was assigned to one of two portals, one leading back to the street for a return home and the other leading to a large enclosed yard. Tiger and Myung Ho were directed toward the latter.

Others designated to the same site were as young as the two boys, or older up to, perhaps, the mid-forties in age. No one had a head full of white hair. No one walking with a limp or stooped in any way was led toward this group.

Before long, the boys and men in the yard were ordered to follow the lead soldier to a new site. The band was shepherded by soldiers bearing arms—an ominous sight and one their Mothers had clearly pointed out would be indicative of their being held as captives.

They were led to Wangshimni located several miles away. There, they were roughly ushered into a large enclosure already filled with other men and boys, all milling anxiously about.

"Clearly, we are captives and would likely be taken North to serve in their military, or to be relegated to slave labor camps," Myung Ho and Tiger agreed in whispers to each other. Speaking in undertones while stealing furtive glances around the compound to assess the dimension of their challenge, they agreed to seek a means of escape soon after dusk.

Men and boys were still being brought into the enclosure throughout the rest of the day.

Apparently, the wire fence had only recently been installed as it was bare of grass with newly turned dirt under the wire stakes, both observed.

Myung Ho and Tiger slowly edged backward towards the fence, moving slowly so as not to attract any attention. By now the sun was beginning to set. The captives were getting thirsty and hungry, growing increasingly restless, raising the background noise. This made it much easier for the boys to reach the fence.

Once there, both boys began to pull at the fence to displace the webbed prongs and stakes, one at a time. To do so, they had to dig with their fingers, working around each stake reaching down more than eight or nine inches. Their nails filled with dirt and grit, but they kept on.

Several of the boys and men nearby noticed their maneuvers, understood quickly, and joined in. Tiger and Myung Ho whispered to them to be especially careful not to arouse notice by the soldiers and to keep their actions and movements to a minimum, in synchrony with the movements of the crowd.

Finally, a sufficient number of stakes had been freed to allow a portion of the fence to be bent high enough upward to allow a person to slide under to the other side. Still, no one dared to slip through.

When the sunlight faded, the compound was illuminated with a searchlight perched on an elevated guard post. Light swept the crowded enclosure periodically solely to allow the armed Communist soldiers to scan the captive group, not for the benefit of the captured throng.

When it had gotten sufficiently dark, following the latest swath of the searchlight, the few who participated in the digging of the stakes rolled under or over the distorted wire fence, one by one, and quickly and quietly crept away from the compound. Each of the escapees remained quiet, not making a sound. The droning sounds from the hungry and thirsty crowd milling about provided sufficient cover.

Yard by yard, the several who had escaped made their way further and further from the compound, headed toward different parts of the city of Seoul.

Myung Ho and Tiger stuck together, moving from one site to the next safe spot, keeping in the shadows, away from the few cars and streetlights, headed towards their homes on Iksundong.

Finally, they reached the yard of the Elementary School both had attended near their homes. Carefully, they crossed the yard without encountering anyone and immediately proceeded to Myung Ho Kim's house, as advised earlier by their Mothers.

Tiger's Mother had agreed that Dr. Kim's house would be a safer place to hide the boys as her house would be a natural target for the Communists in the event of a search for teenage escapees intended for their military or slave labor camps.

Watching anxiously for the boys, Mrs. Kim hurried out to greet them as soon as she heard the sound of their front gate closing. Quickly, she ushered them into the house even before hugging each one, once they were in. She prepared a quick meal for them and soon after they had wolfed down their share, she led them into the closet of the main hall. From there, they reached the attic after dislodging a ceiling board and climbing up a short portable ladder.

Mrs. Kim brought water in a glass bottle, food, bowls and utensils, blankets and other essentials, including a bucket for their waste, for them to camp for the night and the coming days.

Furthermore, she instructed them that three knocks signaled the way was clear for the delivery of their meals. One loud knock followed by a series of quiet taps signaled danger, at which point they were to keep quiet until three knocks signaled all clear. Should they need anything, they were to knock once followed by a minute or more before repeating with only one knock.

With that, Mrs. Kim withdrew the ladder after replacing the ceiling board and shut the closet door. She closed her eyes in a quiet prayer and crossed herself, pleading in her heart for the continued safety of her son and Tiger.

Soon thereafter, she notified Tiger's Mother and the women hugged each other in gratitude for the return of their sons. Mrs. Kim and her family were Catholics and she instinctively thanked God, the Son, and the Holy Ghost for their safe return, making the sign of the cross again as she had done innumerable times since her son had departed with Tiger to answer the Communists' edict.

Mrs. Kang was used to Mrs. Kim's religious gestures and she nodded her head in agreement. She promised to bring articles of clothing, bedding and food for her own son as soon as possible and left assured that Tiger was safe for now.

Like a continuing adventurous saga, the boys quickly adapted to life in the attic, learning to listen with their ears pinned to the floor of the attic for sounds below. A small window allowed sufficient light through for reading books for part of the day. They even became accustomed to holding off the use of the outhouse until stipulated times when the coast was absolutely clear.

Periodically, Tiger's Mother would come over to see him, reassuring him that everyone else at home was alright, that though his Father had not yet returned, he would in time. In this manner, they remained hiding in the attic for nearly two and a half months.

During this time, Myung Ho and Tiger discussed a range of issues from the fate of Tiger's Father, to the last assignments at school, and the likelihood of being picked for the hockey and soccer teams for the next season at Kyonggi High School.

As time passed, Myung Ho raised the question of the origins of the universe, the world and Man, the concept of God, the fate of Man after death, and so forth. Myung Ho divulged his belief in Catholicism to Tiger, who listened with quiet interest.

Tiger gave his own answers to the question of the origins of the universe, where he thought he had information. At other times, Tiger joined in heated debate with Myung Ho, when issues were not clear to him. Tiger believed in a God who watched over his ancestors, ensuring their existence even after death in the spirit world and these very ancestors contributed to the well being of their current family's status, promising safety, good health and prosperity. These teachings of Confucius underlined the way he was raised and his outlook on life.

Each spoke sincerely, asking penetrating questions and waiting patiently for reprieve from the prolonged incarceration they were undergoing in the attic of Dr. Kim's house at Iksun-dong in Seoul.

One day in September at an unexpected hour, there were three distinct knocks on the wall below. Myung Ho and Tiger pushed the ceiling board away and peered down.

It was Myung Ho's father who told the boys to descend from the attic immediately, which they did promptly.

They were told that a house-to-house search was being conducted by the Communists for men and boys not reporting for military or slave labor conscription. Because the attic was a sure place for them to search, they were to hide elsewhere. Their porch or veranda had a narrow storage area below it. This, the doctor believed would be a better, safer site for them. However, it was not as roomy as the attic and would require them to crouch. Still, it would be far safer, he said, and would not likely be searched.

And so, the boys moved to the new site.

The routine continued as before except there was no room to sit up or stand like there had been in the attic and no window existed to let any light in. Now, they had only room enough to crawl and turn over. The cramped condition of their bondage stressed them immeasurably, but they endured.

About this time, the tide of the war had begun to change. After withdrawing to the south towards Taegu and establishing the Pusan Perimeter, the UN troops had successfully landed at Inchon during a narrow window of time between major tidal shifts of the sea on the 15th of September. With constant barrage of firearms, Allied forces were fighting to recapture Seoul and to cut off the supply route for the Communists fighting in the Pusan Perimeter area.

The populace had some knowledge of these circumstances and nearly everyone was aware of the encroachment of the Allies on Seoul. Even the boys had been informed of the Allied landing and movements. Now, they could hear the sounds of battle again and each was excited about the coming reprieve to his physical and social confinement.

Suddenly one day, they heard and felt the pounding of booted feet on the veranda above them. It was a frightening sound, portending dire consequences as Tiger was reminded of the time the Commies came to take his Father away.

Crouching low to avoid hitting the overhanging beam off to his right, Tiger made his way toward the right, dragging himself forward with his forearms braced on the floor of the narrow space built between the overlying porch and the ground.

Listening carefully, he heard a man shouting demandingly and loudly, "Where are the men of this house? Someone fired flares and signals from this section to signal the enemy! They must be hiding somewhere in this house! Where are they? Tell us now or we'll beat it out of you!"

Without any further notice, one of the soldiers hit Mrs. Kim's somewhere on her body with the butt of his rifle and followed this with a loud smack of his hand, also somewhere on her body, probably her cheek, from the sounds Tiger heard.

She cried out loudly in pain. Immediately there arose the cries of her young sons, three of them, probably clinging to their mother's skirt, Tiger thought from the muffled sounds he heard.

Where was the good doctor wondered Tiger? He could hear Myung Ho's three younger brothers crying in alarm at the beating of their mother and the trauma she withstood. The terror of the intrusion by the strangely dressed, hostile men bearing rifles, shouting demands and striking their mother, must have caused them to cling to her skirt and holler in utter panic, he thought recalling the earlier episode at his own home with his young sisters when Father was taken away.

"No one has done any such thing! We don't know what you are talking about! And, my husband is not here. He went to work at Seoul National Hospital helping your injured men. There's no one here but my little sons and myself," sobbed the mother, as she must have rubbed her cheek and then embraced her sons to protect them from any possible blows, Tiger imagined.

Oh, so the doctor is not around. He went to work already, thought Tiger. Unbeknown to Tiger and Myung Ho, at that very moment, her husband and his brother were hiding in the very attic above the main closet, which they themselves had previously occupied for months.

Myung Ho's mother had lied about her husband's absence, but would sustain other blows if necessary to protect her loved ones, not only her husband, but her elder son, her brother-in-law currently in hiding with her husband, and also her neighbors' son, Tiger, as well as the little ones she was hugging tightly, as she crouched down low and gathered them in her arms.

Ordinarily, the surgeon would have been away at the hospital in surgery. However this morning, his brother, who had been in hiding elsewhere, had suddenly appeared. Vacating his previous hiding site because of the house-to-house search, he had made his way to the surgeon's home. Apparently, he had not reported to the authorities as ordered earlier, fearing enforced conscription. He had remained out-of-sight, first elsewhere, and now in the surgeon's attic, just as his nephew Myung Ho and Tiger had done and were still doing.

Sensing imminent danger to himself as well, the surgeon had impulsively joined his brother, climbing into the attic when news of the house-to-house search had come from a network of neighbors looking out for each other. Neither had anything to do with the supposed subversive activity of sending off signals to the Allies, but the brother had not reported to the authorities as ordered earlier and would thereby be highly suspected by the Communists.

The soldiers drew back the sliding doors of the closets that banked two sides of the room and pulled the contents of clothes, books, and pillows out, tossing them towards the center of the room, searching for men.

One of them noticed that the ceiling panel in the closet leading to the space where the doctor and his brother were hiding was slightly askew. He shouted to the others, who quickly joined him. Together they tore off the sliding door to the closet, breaking open the ceiling.

"Come out, or we'll shoot you dead right where you are! Keep your arms up, understand?"

With that, the husband of the woman, the surgeon Kim, and his brother responded, calling out in desperation, "OK, OK, hold your fire, we're coming down, right now!"

Each jumped down from the ceiling onto the floor of the closet and immediately raised his arms up high, looking fearfully at the captors.

"What do you want with us anyway, what have we done? I am a surgeon at Seoul National University and I have provided surgical care to your injured comrades," said the surgeon.

"Are there any others? Who else is hiding? Where are they?" demanded the officer with the non-commissioned men, all bearing arms and looking fiercely angry.

"There's no one else," said the surgeon. The look on his face together with his wife's frightened look told the officer otherwise.

"Search everywhere," the officer ordered his men.

They proceeded to search the entire house. One of the soldiers looked under the veranda. Spotting the enclosed storage area, he pulled open the latched door, exposing the boys.

"Aaahah, no one else, huh! Look what I have found! Now, should I shoot you here or will you come out with your hands up!" he teased, menacingly.

In addition to the search of the area for those responsible for sending off lighted signals to the Allies, the soldiers were also rounding up eligible men for the Democratic People's Republic of Korea for either military conscription or use as slave labor crews. They waited for the boys to jump down from the crawl space.

Once the captives were together, the soldiers barked at them, demanding to know if they had lighted flares and sent signals. They wanted to know who the signals were meant for, where the enemy receiving the signals was located, and so forth.

With each denial, the soldiers struck the captives on the head or face with their fists. Frustrated with their captives, they roughed the men and the two boys. Then pushing them apart they set to handicap each prisoner. First, they wrenched one arm over the opposite shoulder while the other arm was forcibly bent and placed against the back before binding both wrists together over one shoulder with rope. Then, with wrists linked together in this most wrenching position, the prisoners were tethered together, one to the other in a human chain with additional rope. Finally, the soldiers led the band of prisoners towards the door by means of a rifle butt braced against the back of the lead man.

Out onto the streets of Seoul they were led, down the road and up the next several streets, across town to the same wired area designated for men who were being rounded up in the Communists' latest sweep of the capital city of South Korea.

Tiger and Myung Ho could not believe they were back in the compound they had successfully escaped from a couple of months before! Now, they were tethered together with Myung Ho's father and uncle!

There were many other men and boys all looking grim— grimmer than the look the crowd wore the time before at this same place, thought Tiger. To boot, some were tethered together with rope like they were and some looked as though they had been beaten from the blood streaks across their faces and blood stains on their clothes. Everyone looked ominously frightened and a pervasive sense of dread could be felt everywhere one turned.

Throughout this ordeal, the sounds of encroaching gunfire had returned after an absence of nearly three months. In fact, active fighting was now going on at the southern limits of Seoul.

Where were the Allies? How could we be in such a circumstance considering the progress the Allies were supposed to have made! Had there been another turn of events to rally the Communists? Will we be dragged to the north, imprisoned, or tortured and killed, each of the captives wondered?

CHAPTER 4: INCARCERATION AND FREEDOM

Once in the compound, the tethers binding the prisoners were not removed, but the captors left them and walked off.

The captured from Dr. Kim's home clustered together with surgeon Kim verbally calming his son and Tiger. Soon his brother gained what little leverage there was to be had to turn around and was engaged in conversation with other men and boys in small cowering groups near by, asking them how and where they were caught.

It was nearing dusk and fires could be seen off in the distance to the west and south while both gunfire and cannon fire could be heard to be encroaching ever closer, though intermittently, along the western borders.

As the day darkened even further with the sounds of battle increasing in intensity, the Communist soldiers returned to surgeon Kim and his group. They dragged the surgeon upright and re-interrogated him about the signals he was supposed to have sent, demanding to know the nature of the information transmitted, the recipient of the message, his involvement with one political group or another, and so forth. With each negative answer or denial of involvement, Kim was struck on the face or body by the lead interrogator using both fists and hands.

The brutality of the interrogation alarmed the surgeon's brother. Fearing that the repeated beatings could damage his brother irreversibly and even lead to brutal trauma to others in the small group, he launched on a campaign to engage them in what he knew best how to do, carrying on in conversation. First, he jokingly suggested that he not be deprived of such good treatment. One of the soldiers immediately slapped him on the face.

Undaunted, he continued to speak, commenting on a wide variety of non-political issues, first with one of the attackers, then with another, and another, and then back to the first one again. He talked incessantly, neglecting to keep silent when ordered to, and taking a punch or a slap here and there as the captors were wont to do in response to his constant chatter. Because of his unceasing small talk, the captors relinquished further interrogation or beating of the surgeon, concentrating instead on his brother and trying to get him to divulge various bits of the information they were seeking.

All the while, the sounds of battle grew louder and louder, indicative of the continuing encroachment of the U.S. and South Korean forces to the prisoner holding site. Now, the darkness was interrupted with bright flares that accompanied the blasts, exposing the evening scene.

Minutes later, the sounds of battle indicated the opposing forces were virtually upon the compound. The looks on the captors changed starkly from anger and rage to that of alarm and panic.

The captors shouted orders to get ready to dispose of the prisoners and to be alert for orders to move to the rear. A few shots were heard together with loud pleading voices and shouts followed by groans from groups of captives within the compound, who were the initial victims of an intended wholesale slaughter. With a sudden jerk on the lead man, one of the captors of surgeon Kim's group pulled the tethered prisoners upright, altogether at one time. Stepping back to target them with a gun that he withdrew from a holster at his side, he was about ready to begin the slaughter of this group of prisoners.

Suddenly, a loud burst of cannon-fire exploded nearby accompanied by a bright illumination, announcing the undeniable presence of the opposing forces in the immediate area.

Temporarily shaken, the lead captor shouted loudly to his men, "Let's go! All of you let's go!"

Without further ado, each Communist soldier immediately followed the leader out of the area, running, headed north.

Unbelievably, the would-be slaughterers had left without completing the grisly task they had intended to accomplish just a few moments before!

With hearts racing all the way, everyone felt immediate, instantaneous relief!

The two boys could hardly believe the sequence of events in the last hours on this day, the 24th of September in 1950. The hiding for months since the fall of Seoul with only intermittent, brief periods of relief was, perhaps, finally over. The terror of their capture and their survival by the miraculous timing of the arrival of the U.S. and South Korean forces at the moment of their imminent execution would forever be etched in their minds and hearts.

The culmination of their capture was for all four a truly religious experience with God personally intervening upon their behalf to eventuate their rescue. How else could such a near-death experience have turned into a routing of the enemy and a reprieve for each?

They were humbled beyond words and there was no way to stem the flow of tears of joy streaming from their eyes. The surgeon, his son, and his brother repeatedly praised God, thanking Him for intervening and seeing to their survival.

Tiger listened through his tears, very impressed with their devotion to God. His family had come from a long line of people who honored their ancestors and lived by a code of ethics akin to Confucianism. They were not Buddhists, but were acquainted with Buddhist customs. Following the withdrawal of the Japanese, Christian precepts, particularly those promulgated by the Catholics, were increasingly being spread and widely accepted. Still, no one in the Kang family had become a Christian, as of yet.

The surgeon expressed gratefulness to his talkative brother who kept the captors at bay with his constant chatter, distracting the soldiers long enough for the home forces to reach the prisoner compound. Otherwise, they might have all been killed, or the surgeon would have been beaten to near-death, they all agreed. (This experience was to affect each of the captives in the profoundest ways in the years to come.)

They untied each other quickly, rubbing the bruises on their wrists, arms, faces and other parts that were brutally struck in the course of their captivity. They huddled together as an armed force reached the compound, everyone watching carefully to be sure the force was not composed of retreating Communist stragglers.

Once they recognized that the troops were friendly, the prisoners greeted them with loud shouts of hurrahs and hand clapping. The former captives related the horror of their capture and the drama of the last few minutes of their incarceration to the liberators, whether they understood Korean or not, thanking them over and over again for the timeliness of their rescue.

Sadly, the soldiers discovered the bodies of the several men and boys who had been shot, and ordered the rest of the saved to see to their proper burial at one end of the compound.

Because it was night already and Allied troops were in movement, the survivors were advised to remain within the compound until morning. The soldiers bid them farewell and continued the task of pushing the enemy troops of the Democratic People's Republic of Korea further north.

All night long, the sounds of firearms could be heard and the evening was lit with the near continuous bursting of explosives. Before long however, gradually, the intensity of the battle sounds lessened, somewhat. No one slept as they watched the fireworks into the dawn. With the approach of full daylight by which time the sounds of war had moved considerably north, Dr. Kim indicated it was time to return home.

Walking carefully to avoid being mistaken for the enemy by other Allied soldiers moving northward, Tiger could hardly believe that the recent ordeal was over. He would not have to hide again. Considering all he had undergone in the recent months, the loss of his Father, hiding for months, and the most recent trauma of capture, incarceration, and the threat of death, he did not know how much more he could take. He was coming to the realization that his Father might not return within the immediately foreseeable future. Because of his Father's political activities, he would not be released he was sure, especially considering the manner in which the Communists dealt with innocent civilians such as the Kims and himself. Yet, Tiger hoped they would see the benefit to their own Communist society of his medical skills and allow him to live. Rumors were rampant about the skilled being taken to the Democratic People's Republic of Korea to fill the needs of the Communists. While no word had come from anyone about his Father's status, he would force himself to believe that his Father was still alive and would someday return, hopefully sooner than later.

Tiger thought about his Mother and her grief over the loss of her husband. Surely, she must have learned of the capture of her eldest son by now. At least, she would be consoled by his safe return, he thought, breaking into a warm smile.

With that, he had an urge to race ahead, but kept in line with the Kims instead, walking slowly and carefully so as not to arouse any suspicion on the part of the defenders of his country, who could be seen moving in the reverse direction with rifles fixed with bayonets, glancing at everyone for any signs of opposition.

CHAPTER 5: MOTHER, OH, MOTHER!

Before long, the group approached Iksun-dong, the street where the families Kang and Kim lived close to each other—families of two physicians, one an internist and the other a surgeon.

The men were close and their wives were good friends. The Kangs had four daughters, one older than Tiger by two years, and three others who were younger than Tiger, each about two years apart from one another. Tiger's younger brother, Pyo, was about the same age as Kim's middle son and they often played together. Although their yards did not adjoin and each was fenced in, their sons had found ready ways of overcoming these barriers to interact in a multitude of ways in the years and months before June 25th.

As the group approached their homes, there was a distinct pall that hung in the air, not entirely ascribable to the smoky atmosphere hovering over the entire city of Seoul. Hardly any civilian movement was noticeable in the neighborhood and while the sounds of war could still be heard, it was distant and the area was strangely quiet.

Tiger thanked the Kims for all they had done for him and bowed to them as he approached the gate to his home. Dr. Kim patted him on the shoulder and Myung Ho promised to be in touch real soon to continue some of their activities.

Stepping beyond the gate, he had an unexplained sense of foreboding, for the area surrounding the house had never been so quiet. Even after his Father had been taken away by the Communists, his younger brother and sisters made a certain clamor that was audible immediately outside the house inside the front gate.

Quickly, he let himself into the house and called out, "Mother, I'm back, where are you?"

Out of the back rooms, his younger siblings came forth rather slowly and with evident caution. Neither his older sister Ok Im, nor his Mother was with them.

Recognizing him, his younger sisters rushed forward, crying out loudly, "It's Kun oh-pa (Big Brother). You're back!"

"We were so worried about you, knowing that the awful Communists had captured you and all the Kims. Oh, oh, how can we tell you what has happened to our beloved Mother? How can we?" they cried. Quickly drawing back, they began to whimper and cry, now shedding real tears.

"What's this? What are you saying? Tell me, where is Mother and where is Ok Im?" asked Tiger.

"Oh Oh-pa (Brother), Ok Im is up at Ui-dong with Grandfather. But, yesterday the Communist soldiers arrested Mother, our cousin, and his wife with her infant strapped on her back, dragging them out of the house. We do not know why they were taken away and where they were taken to."

"And, Mother has not yet returned!" they blurted, each letting out a cry.

"What are you saying? What are you saying? How can that be? Don't you know where they took Mother? Where's To-oma and the other helpers in the house?"

With the commotion, To-oma appeared, as well as the other household servants. "Yes, your Mother, your cousin and his wife with her baby strapped on her back were dragged away by the enemy soldiers," they said wringing their hands, reinforcing what his siblings had just told him.

Apparently, Ok Im had gone to Tiger's maternal Grandfather's home at Ui-dong and had been gone for several days. Neither she nor Grandfather had yet been informed as these events only took place a day ago, they told him.

"We've got to find Mother. I'll go to Uncle's house to find out more and for help," he said.

After consoling his siblings and promising to return as soon as possible, he walked out of the house, passed through the front gate and headed for his Uncle Choi's house.

Tiger reached Dr. Han Woong Choi's home and was met by Han Woong's sister-in law, who had been staying there since the outbreak of the war along with her two children, who were Tiger's cousins.

The elder of her two children, Hak Joo, was a number of years younger than Tiger. He and Tiger had spent many happy weekend and summer days together at their Grandfather's place at Ui-dong, splashing in the brook, shaking down the chestnut trees for nuts, and challenging each other at the board game called pa-duk, all under the watchful eye of their Grandfather, Yukdang or Choi Nam Sun, a well-known literary great in Korea.

Hak Joo's mother shouted with joy on seeing Tiger and hugged him briefly. She had heard of his capture and had feared the worse. Tears streamed down her face as she pulled back from him to look to see if he had any evidence of abuse on his face.

Tiger immediately asked, "Where is my Mother? Do you know where she is and what has happened to her?"

Shaken, his Aunt ushered him into Han Woong's home, sat him down on a chair and told him that his Mother was arrested along with his cousin and his cousin's wife, who was carrying their infant son, by marauding Communist troops as the Allies were approaching Seoul. No one knew where they had been taken to, but his Aunt felt that they would all return shortly as the Allies were retaking Seoul. A little patience was all that was needed for his Mother to find her way back, she reassured him.

Her own brother-in-law, the good Dr. Han Woong Choi, had not returned home from Seoul National University Hospital. They believed he was still working, but it had been three days already without a word from him. Surely, he must be alright, just simply unable to reach home, she reassured Tiger.

Bewildered, perplexed and extremely exhausted, Tiger wanted to believe her and so left for home, prepared to wait a bit longer to see his beloved Mother to return safe and unharmed.

The sounds of battle seemed to be further and further away as the Communists steadily retreated. To-oma and the others managed the family, fixed dinner and fed everyone. By evening, Mother had not returned and there was still no word of Dr. Han Woong Choi's whereabouts. Exhausted, Tiger fell into a restless sleep, tossing and turning as though his body yearned for the hardness of the hiding spaces to which he had become accustomed instead of the firm comfort of his sleeping pad. Fleeting visions of angry, hostile men armed with rifles threatening him and striking him with a blow here and another there, interrupting his search for his Father and his Mother in a hodge-podge of dreamy episodes plagued him throughout the night.

Barely rested, the next day, Tiger began his search for his Mother again. He canvassed the neighborhood, knocking and inquiring about any possible witnessing of the arrest or knowledge of the whereabouts of his Mother, his cousin, and his cousin's wife and baby.

No one had seen them. Ominously, one of the men he met told him about a group of people, including women and children, having been killed by a rag-tag army of Communist stragglers in a field nearby.

"If you can't find them, you ought to consider the unfortunate possibility that they might have been included in the group that was killed," he had suggested with a sad, sad look on his haggard face.

After another futile day of waiting to no avail, with great sadness Tiger finally decided he would have to find and check out the site mentioned by the man the day before.

He walked to the open field indicated by the man as the site of the killing spree. It was the field where he had regularly played soccer with the other boys of the neighborhood.

As he approached the familiar field, he was alarmed to find a section of the previously grass-covered ground exposed with dirt covering what looked like a newly formed mound. The mound-like formation had not been there before he went into hiding some months before and it was clear the dirt had only recently been turned over. And, it had the ominous appearance of a burial site.

"I must find my Mother, dead or alive. I cannot go on without knowing what has become of her!" he said to his Aunt, as he bolstered himself and began scooping the dirt with his hands.

His Aunt had come along with him on this search. Seeing that the mound resembled a burial site, she cried within herself not only for the likely trauma to Tiger and his siblings in finding her there, but also for herself as she and Tiger's Mother were not only related by marriage but were very close friends. Unable to delay Tiger's intent to seek out the identity of the buried, she pleaded with him to hold off the digging until she had returned with a shovel.

Tiger nodded, promising to await her return. Apprehensively, he sat on the ground beside the mound. Looking up towards the sky, he hoped and, yes, prayed to his ancestors that he would not find his Mother amongst the buried.

He gratefully took the shovel his Aunt brought back shortly thereafter and began to remove the dirt from the top of the mound. It did not take long before he uncovered the first body, a lady, obviously the last one to be slaughtered, his logic told him.

Reeling from the stench of rotting human flesh, he peered at her face. It appeared to be that of a middle-aged woman who died in terror, for her eyes were still open and her mouth was wide agape as though she had not finished screaming. It was horrible! Her throat was slit from ear to ear, exposing the tendons, air ducts, and vessels and everything was covered with dried blood, now fully brownish-black, and dirt.

He gently laid her back and proceeded to uncover the next body. No, it was not his Mother, he said to himself. He worked his way down, uncovering others. In all, there must have been several dozens of corpses in the grave. By now, the stench no longer bothered him. With each corpse, he searched the face intently, looking for his Mother. None looked like her, none at all!

"See," he said with a peculiar sense of relief to his Aunt, "My Mother is not amongst these dead! So, she must still be alive!"

After a moment of elation because he had not found his Mother, a deep sadness overcame him as he wondered where his Mother might have been taken to and what could have become of her.

Relieved after his fruitless search, he returned to the task of returning each body back into the uncovered mass grave. With each corpse, he took more time to stare at the face. Now he recognized the local herbalist here, the man at the post office there, the wife of Mr. Lee there, and so forth.

Nearing the end of his gruesome task, he looked at a woman with an infant strapped on her back. He was startled to see that the woman resembled the wife of his cousin. He had not recognized her before, having focused solely on finding his Mother. Indeed, she was his cousin's wife and now he even could see that the infant was, in fact, his cousin's baby! The distortions resulting from the manner of killing together with the blood and dirt conspired to disguise their true identities.

Alarmed, he looked carefully at the face of the man under the woman's body. It was his cousin! With great foreboding, he looked at the only remaining body yet to be returned to the grave, the first one he had uncovered.

"Oh, Mother! Mother! Mother!" he cried. "It is you! I did not recognize you before, but it is you! How could I?" he sobbed as he laid her head back gently on the ground.

"They ripped your neck from ear to ear and your dying face changed so, I did not recognize my own sweet, dear Mother! You were the first one I uncovered. You must have been the last to be killed."

"Mother! Oh, Mother! It is you!"

He sobbed and sobbed, not to be consoled by anything or anyone for several minutes.

A few minutes later, his Aunt closed in and held Tiger by the shoulders. She too, saw her own sister-in-law, the beloved wife of Dr. Kang, the mother of two sons and four daughters, the only daughter of the great intellectual and patriot, Choi Nam Sun or Yukdang, dead by virtue of a slashing wound from ear to ear that severed the vessels and laryngeal tubes of her neck. How filled with terror she must have been at the end, with her eyes wide open even in death and her mouth agape! How awful a death! And the pain and horror of this moment for Tiger! she thought, as she brushed away her own tears.

After all the tears his body could muster had been released, Tiger looked up to his Aunt. His Mother's body lay before him, gruesome in manner of death but wholly beloved by her son who could grieve no further—now fully spent.

In full sympathy, his Aunt quickly took hold of the situation and instructed Tiger to withhold her body and that of his cousin, along with his cousin's wife and child for burial at a private site.

Sorrowfully, he nodded his head in agreement, but asked her how all of what she proposed was to be accomplished.

"Leave it to me," she assured him. "Now, return home and ready yourself for the task that lies ahead."

With that, Tiger slowly arose from the pile of dirt, wiped his face of the dripping wetness with the sleeves of his shirt, streaking his face with dirt, and stumbling forward, headed for home.

Together with help mustered from sympathetic neighbors and friends, including the surgeon Kim and his family, his Aunt oversaw the availability of blankets for use as makeshift pallets. The bodies were brought to the house on Iksun-dong and arrangements were made by his Aunt to place them in proper garments before laying them in wooden coffins, which she had somehow or other arranged to be built.

A gathering of only a few neighbors and relatives, including Dr. Han Woong Choi's family with the good doctor conspicuously absent, sat, wept, and consoled the children, remembering the goodness of Mother Kang and her kindness to all, most recently extending her kindness to those who unfortunately were killed along with her.

His Grandfather, Choi Nam San, was also not there for his only daughter's funeral. No one could be dispatched to the northern outskirts of Seoul where he lived as it was still within the line of fighting, too risky an area to traverse.

There was no feasting as would have been done per custom during earlier times. This was all that could be done at this point during the war.

The coffins were taken to the nearest vacant site they could find and buried without further fanfare. No markers were possible and only knowledge that the beloved had been mourned and buried remained in Tiger's memory and heart.

After the burial, Tiger returned to Iksun-dong with his siblings. To-oma oversaw their immediate needs and after a few days saw to the transmission of the sad news to Grandfather and the return of Tiger's elder sister back home when the Communists were well routed back North, above the 38th parallel.

Meanwhile, the whereabouts of their uncle, Dr. Han Woong Choi had become a matter of grave concern to everyone. Apparently, the retreating Communists had forced medical personnel at Seoul National University Hospital to march as captives, for utilization of their services in the North.

Remarkably, after a month of capture and a painful slow trek to the North, Allied paratroopers had landed near by the marching line of prisoners and successfully dealt with their captors. Following the fracas, Dr. Han Woong Choi and the others were freed to make their way safely back home.

And so, a month after the good doctor had disappeared, he returned, worn and shaken, but alive and unhurt.

Tiger's Aunt oversaw the proper stocking of their kitchen to enable them to survive for a few days. Everyone was quiet and inactive. The absence of first, their Father, then their Mother, left each with a sense of abandonment, fear of the future, and a frank sense of depression, not knowing what to do next, or how to do whatever needed to be done.

They had been raised in a privileged family where hired help saw to the tasks of the daily chores. Since the fall of Seoul, their household help had diminished considerably. After their Father was arrested, their Mother had only two others beside To-oma to assist her, where she had several others before. Now that their Mother was gone, who would oversee the household?

Ok Im, the eldest, was in her last year of high school at the outbreak of the war. She had never prepared an entire meal before. The household had been fully staffed with paid and unpaid caretakers (relatives) providing for the family and a roster of visiting distant family members, many of whom frequently stayed on for weeks. With the loss of both parents,

Ok Im's challenges were to quickly assume the role of cook, housekeeper, and supervisor of her younger siblings with some help from Tiger.

Uncle Han Woong, his wife, and his sister-in-law, Hak Joo's mother, frequently dropped off food items and money. Their Father's medical office and clinic were closed. Relatives advised them to sell their contents and to rent these sites to another physician and to the many who were seeking alternative homes as a result of the destruction of their houses.

And so, the surviving members of the family Kang were forced to make temporary adjustments for the loss of both parents and the conditions of a war, which raged back and forth, wreaking havoc on the inhabitants of South Korea, especially on those dwelling around it's capital, Seoul.

Among the changes they underwent was a reduction of meals, not only in size and variety of content, but also in number from three or more in the past to just two a day. Lunch was forgone, as there was not the means to purchase the items.

To make ends meet, Tiger quickly learned that most of the Allied soldiers smoked cigarettes and that they were willing to pay for packs or individual cigarettes for a sum good enough for a satisfying meal to a half-starved Korean. One could purchase a whole carton from a black marketer and reap a small profit by selling the cigarettes, one at a time.

Humiliated, but in desperation, Tiger tried this for a brief period, using his profit to bring home the bean sprouts and tofu for a soup to eat with rice they still had in storage. Once in a while, there was even enough for some dried fish, but never enough for meat. He and the rest of the family developed a special craving for meat, which went unmet for long periods of time.

As the weather cooled, coal and other fuels were in short supply. Having to alter their mode of living with the meager resources available was made worse by not having sources for the bare necessities of living available for purchase.

Meanwhile, the battle continued on and on.

CHAPTER 6: EVACUATION TO THE SOUTH

Allied forces continued their efforts to recapture Seoul. The brilliant strategy embarked by General Douglas MacArthur to land at Inchon during a narrow window of time allowable by the widely varying tidal movements of the Yellow Sea had led the Allies to a timely victory, cutting off the Communists' supply lines to their troops south of Seoul pressing along the Pusan perimeter. The enemy forces around Seoul were being routed and now the Allied troops were chasing them beyond the 38th parallel, nearing the Yalu River.

Then, on November 25th a new element changed the balance of the fighting. Hordes of Chinese Communist soldiers crossed the Yalu, surprising and outnumbering the Allied forces. News of the incursion of the Chinese and the subsequent evacuation of Allied forces by the sea at Hungnam rapidly circulated throughout the world even reaching the suffering citizens of Seoul.

As the Allies were being routed and the line of battle was rapidly moving south again, a decision was made by Tiger's relatives for Tiger, his older sister Ok Im and the sister immediately below him, Duk Im, and his brother Pyo to evacuate along with Dr. Han Woong Choi's family and his Father, Choi Nam Sun, to Taegu, near Pusan. Tiger's experiences, the loss of both of his parents, Han Woong's encounter with the Communists and his return following the intervention of the Allied paratroopers left no doubt about the matter. Han Woong's wife had come from the city of Taegu and family members would provide them living space. Tiger's two youngest siblings, who were under ten years of age, would remain behind in Seoul under the care of their Grandmother, Choi Nam Sun's wife.

It was mid-December in 1950 when the family members bid each other farewell and looked for a means to escape to the south. Allied troops were hastily being moved to the same region to make another stand. Train cars were filled with wounded soldiers being evacuated to the field hospitals already in the south. Only the roofs of the rail cars were available for the civilians, who gladly clambered aboard with their individual bundles, grateful for the opportunity to ride away from the encroaching battle lines instead of walking the hundreds of miles along damaged and sometimes mined roads.

Exposure to the cold was made worse by the force of the train's movement against the air, dissipating body heat, dropping temperatures further despite the clothing worn by the civilians riding atop the cars. In fact, frost actually bit the extremities of the riders. Tiger's toes felt frozen, so cold all pain subsided, replaced by numbness that even touching and rubbing with his cold hands could not re-warm or stimulate. The effect of this insult was to last long after the trauma of this ride with the circulation to his toes seemingly forever insufficient and inadequate, no matter how warm the actual skin temperature to these appendages.

The train moved slowly, hauling well in excess of its usual capacity. It also stopped here and there for troop exchanges and refueling with coal. After a couple of days, the train came to a halt at Taegu Station. Everyone gladly got off with his individual bundle. Many were hobbling because of their long exposure to the cold in a cramped position, but all seemed relieved at having reached a safe haven, however temporary.

The family members gathered their belongings and muddled their way to Han Woong Choi's in-laws. There, after warm greetings were exchanged with great emotions, assignments were made for everyone to use a part of their space as a home base.

It was crowded, to be sure, but everyone was provided for. Tiger and his three siblings shared a room with a maternal aunt of his uncle's wife. There was food enough for all and warmth, both physical and emotional, to share. They had escaped with sufficient casualty to their family to last many life times. Everyone was grateful to have arrived intact, trusting and believing that the two youngest daughters of Dr. and Mrs. Kang and their Grandmother, would not likely be victimized by the Communists, should they reoccupy Seoul.

Before long, it was clear that the influx of so many relatives would set a burden on the resources of Dr. Choi's in-laws. Dr. Choi's wife was fully cognizant of this and quickly set out to seek a means to provide additional resources for the family's living requirements.

Several tours to the market areas and observation of the dietary preferences of the Allied troops on leave had suggested a possibility for a business venture to her. After discussion with her husband and winning his approval, she gathered the family and told them of her plan.

Her brother had a bookstore located on the main street in Taegu. Book sales had not gone well since the outbreak of the war. The bookshelves could be turned around converting the store into a coffee house where tea or coffee could be served with French fried potatoes to hungry Allied troops on leave, she explained. She and the girls would cook and serve, Tiger would take the orders because he spoke some English, and the others would clean and run errands.

Everyone agreed to participate, and it was not long thereafter that Dr. Choi's wife had converted the bookstore into a thriving coffee house. It was conveniently located to attract soldiers on leave with the tantalizing odors emanating from the frying of freshly cut sticks of potatoes in heated pots of fat. Together with a cup of coffee or tea, French fries liberally sprinkled with salt and pepper rapidly became a favorite snack to any American within a smelling distance of the area.

The eatery thrived, bringing everyone of the newly arrived from Seoul a sense of accomplishment and freedom from total dependence on their hosts as they contributed to the maintenance of the household expenses.

Tiger used his English to welcome, invite, and take orders from the customers. Honing his language skills, he soon picked up new words and phrases that servicemen often used without recognizing some to be offensive.

"We serve damn good French Fries!" he would hawk. Encouraging the servicemen strolling around the area to enter their stall, he promised them a god-damn good snack.

Over the next six months, Tiger ran into a number of his former classmates as well as other friends and neighbors from Seoul, who had also moved to the Taegu area, or were moving on to the port city of Pusan after the Chinese had entered the war. With each encounter, he asked about the possible escape of prisoners and whether or not anyone had seen his Father, to no avail.

One day after enjoying the snack, one of the patrons of the coffee shop who was a Korean asked Tiger of his possible interest in working as an interpreter for the 5th U.S. Air Force. That unit was about ready to move from Taegu to Kimpo

Airbase just outside of Seoul. The Allies were beginning to push the Chinese back North and there was need for interpreters to assist them in their communications with their Korean military cohorts. He had appreciated Tiger's ability to entice, welcome and fill the orders of the patrons of the coffee shop in English and considered him a promising candidate. The wage they offered was far greater than anything anyone could have imagined at that time and Tiger viewed this as an opportunity to improve the family's financial state.

Tiger brought the issue to his Grandfather, who agreed that he could pursue the offer. Shortly thereafter, he was interviewed, duly hired, and subsequently moved to Kimpo Airbase with the U.S. 5th Air Force, to work as an interpreter.

During the two months of work at Kimpo, Tiger learned a few other expressions from the American troops, including some four-letter ones without understanding the degree of offensiveness of some of the words and phrases he began to include in his English repertoire. The tour of duty provided free meals through which he was introduced to western fare. It was decidedly different from the hot and spicy dishes he was accustomed to, but there was always plenty to eat including meat of one sort or another almost twice a day. After two months had passed, Tiger returned to Taegu to visit his family.

In the interim, his uncle Han Woong had reopened a part of the bookstore next to the coffee shop. With the continued Allied move towards the Yalu River, residents of the area were once again visiting the bookstore, thereby providing much needed additional financial help.

During this visit, a former classmate, T.J. Yoo, appeared looking for Tiger. T.J.'s family had escaped any casualty from the war. He was working as an attendant on a bus providing service between Taegu and Pusan. His father had purchased the bus following their escape from Seoul to Pusan. Transportation service between Pusan and Taegu was profitable, providing T.J.'s family with funds to augment his father's newly set-up, small medical practice in Pusan.

T.J. invited Tiger to Pusan for a visit. So, Tiger visited the city on the Straits of Japan, where he met many other former Kyonggi buddies. He learned that classes for Kyonggi High School had begun operations in Pusan for those displaced from Seoul using tents as classrooms.

One morning, Tiger joined his classmates to meet some of his old teachers who had also evacuated to Pusan and were now teaching in the tent classrooms. The Principal, the honorable Mang Ju Chun, was overjoyed to see Tiger. He had heard of the tragic circumstances surrounding the loss of both of the student's parents and had been concerned about his whereabouts and wellbeing. Once he had calmed down, Mr. Mang insisted that Tiger return to school to complete his education, making him promise to do so, as soon as possible.

Returning to Taegu to join the family, Tiger told them of the opening of Kyonggi High School in Pusan and of his meeting with the Principal. He raised the matter of completing his education in Pusan with his Uncle and Grandfather.

Both heartily agreed that he should relinquish his current job as soon as possible and complete his education at the makeshift Kyonggi High School in Pusan. Pusan was many miles away from Taegu making it impossible for Tiger to commute on a daily basis.

The question of living arrangements had to be resolved, but first, Tiger returned to Kimpo to formally resign in order to complete his education in Pusan. Though unsure about the details of his support in Pusan, he was determined to complete his education, one way or another.

Shortly thereafter, another former classmate of his, Chung Byung Uk, offered Tiger a place to stay with his family in Pusan. The Chungs had also evacuated from Seoul but had sought refuge in Pusan and had made a successful transition with room enough for Tiger to use.

Gratefully, Tiger moved in with the Chungs and once he was back in school, worked hard to catch up with a year's work in one semester. His performance amazed both classmates and teachers. After only a few months, he completed the year's work and was promoted to the senior year in high school.

At about this time, Seoul was recaptured once again by the Allies and the city was open to the return of nonmilitary personnel. Consequently, Kyonggi High School announced it would be returning to Seoul for the next school session.

This and concern for his younger sisters led Tiger to decide to return to Seoul with his siblings even before the rest of the extended family had decided to return to the capital city of South Korea, Seoul.

Uncle Han Woong, his immediate family and Tiger's Grandfather elected to remain in Taegu for several more months, inasmuch as business was good and they needed to build on their financial resources a bit to gain a foothold in the immediate postwar period to come. They correctly anticipated chaos and financial hardship would ensue in Seoul in the immediate aftermath of the routing of the Communists.

And thus it was that Tiger and his sisters sought to return to Seoul without them.

CHAPTER 7: RETURN, CONVERSION AND A BREAK

In Seoul, Tiger and his siblings found their two younger sisters and their Grandmother together and safe. They had survived the Chinese invasion and the return of the Allied forces to retake Seoul without casualty. Joyful of their safety, they resumed life together. Not long after, the rest of the extended family members and most of their previously displaced friends and neighbors also returned. And by the beginning of April, most schools reopened in Seoul even though the war had not yet officially ended.

As the first-born son of a family now essentially orphaned, though only a senior in high school, Tiger had the taxing responsibility of being the head of the household, looking after their needs and seeing to the allocation of their meager resources.

He learned to eke out their subsistence on the net receipts of the rental payments on the clinic property together with subsidies from Uncle Han Woong against the rising cost of rampant inflation that wreaked havoc with the economy of postwar Korea. He relied heavily on Uncle Han Woong, his wife, and their Grandfather for guidance.

Nevertheless, many a time, decisions had to be made without their input. Little did he know that though these pressures were difficult, such experiences would help him to form personal character traits that were to place him at a decided advantage in the coming future.

By July 1953, armistice negotiations were initiated between the Communist North and the Allied Forces. Without a real settlement, a truce was signed on the 27th of July with the battle lines at the 38th parallel as the de facto boundary between the two halves of the Korean Peninsula.

Despite repatriation and release of prisoners from both sides, Tiger's Father never returned.

Tiger kept the emotionally most unnerving experience, the discovery of his Mother's corpse and the events surrounding it, sequestered in his mind, locked there, not to be reexamined.

However, he could not thwart it's reassertion in disguise mostly, when from time to time, extremely disturbing dreams would occur during sleep when he would shout and holler sounds of terror and anguish that were, fortunately, undecipherable to others. Such occurrences were to recur long, long after his rise to full manhood.

Occasionally, when times were especially hard, Tiger wished that he might have died, instead. He had difficulty reconciling that Myung Ho's God, if he existed, was all loving, or that his ancestors had any power over their destinies, according to Confucius, considering the tragedies he and his family had undergone. Nonetheless, he had to admit that the drama of the miraculous night when the nearby blast saved their small band from execution by their Communist captors could only have occurred because of the intervention of an almighty, caring force—God. The devotion of the Kims had a lasting impression on him. He even wondered whether the Almighty had intervened for *their* sake, not his, and that he might then have only been an indirect beneficiary.

Pondering these issues along with the demands of their very difficult life, he was open to a conversion. Sometime during or shortly after the war, his Grandfather, Choi Nam San, had converted to Catholicism and several others in the family had followed suit. He had heard the basic tenants of the Catholics, but had questions that he could not resolve.

One of his classmates at Kyonggi High School, Peter Lee, occasionally invited Tiger to the Korean Episcopal Church in Seoul to play ping-pong, after school and on the weekends. The table and paddles were available for their use and from time to time, Tiger was free to go along.

Peter's father was an Episcopal Church Warden, who frequently encountered them there. Over the course of time, both Peter and his father would raise spiritual questions for Tiger to consider. Each time, they provided reasonable answers as well as commentary about God, life, death, and the after life. Eventually they succeeded in getting Tiger to attend church services. Before long, the doctrines espoused by the Episcopalians appeared reasonable and much less controversial to Tiger than those espoused by Catholics to Tiger. Consequently, it followed that Tiger could be persuaded to become an Episcopalian.

Peter's father agreed to be his Godfather and selected the name, Andrew, as his baptismal name. Thenceforth, Tiger, now Andrew, became a Christian and began attending Episcopal Church services fairly regularly. He found it personally helpful to pray, convinced that somehow or other, the Almighty existed and heard our desperate pleas. While His ways were not always our ways, He definitely intervened. Else, how could some of the good and life-saving events that transpired in his personal life have come to be? Mere chance could not explain them, no siree! Tiger thought using the military vernacular he had often heard to bring emphasis to his conviction.

Furthermore, he resumed other activities appropriate for his gender, age, and skill. As a youngster, Andrew had learned to skate in the frozen rice paddies up North, during his school break visits to his paternal Grandfather's home. Later, he had excelled as a high school hockey player and was also a fine soccer player on the school team before the Korean War. He was able to resume these activities on the school teams once Kyonggi High School had reopened in Seoul after the capital had been recaptured again.

These activities offered a perfect venue where he could charge, strike and discharge his pent up energies, displacing the raw anger against the loss of his parents and the consequences thereof, which he kept under simmering cover. These were, after all, accepted forms of action helping to quell the reactions he had to the trauma he had experienced. Furthermore, he excelled at these sports, bringing him the pleasures that come with being a winner as well as the much needed psychological relief from the pressures arising upon sustaining the suppression of reactions to his recent tragic experiences.

Soon it was time again for entrance examinations for various colleges to be held throughout Seoul as was the custom, where every college offered it's own exams, for a fee. On a practical basis, one could only apply to a few because of the time and energy involved in the examination processes. In 1953 before he was to graduate from Kyonggi High School, he was faced with the looming dilemma of where to go to college, let alone financing the fees for the entrance examinations as well as the tuition. In order to ensure entrance to a college, wouldn't he have to take tests offered by several colleges, he worried?

Earlier, his Uncle Han Woong had stated simply that he was to apply to Seoul National University to major in medicine. Naturally, he had every intention of following in his Father's footsteps and consequently did not object to his Uncle's pronouncement.

After much consideration, he only applied to one college, Seoul National University, about all he could afford. In the past, he had never experienced nervousness before an examination. Yet, on this occasion, Andrew was peculiarly anxious and nervous. For the first time, he was even sleepless through most of the night and naturally, by morning, he was extremely tired. Undoubtedly, this was due to the cumulative effects of all the stresses he had undergone since the outbreak of the war and his conditioning to perceived threats by heightening reaction.

The examination lasted a couple of days. Whereas he was certain that he had done well in three of the four areas covered, he was not quite sure of his performance in the fourth area. This unsettling anxiety was soon undone when he learned that he had done extremely well, indeed. And so, he was admitted to Seoul National University to study medicine, which would take six years in Korea.

Rental of his Father's clinic to a practicing surgeon and other tenants together with subsidies from his Uncle did not fully provide for the family, especially in the face of a badly deflated Korean currency, the Won, and the rampant rise of inflation. Complicating matters even more, his Grandfather, the patriot and literary genius, Choi Nam San, had suffered a stroke and was now bed-ridden, reducing his Uncle's subsidy.

Consequently, Andrew began to teach English and Mathematics at night to students in need of remedial teaching for a small but much needed fee. This helped them some as any bit of financial help would at this point in their lives. How he was to meet the financial stress of completing his education was not clear, but somehow or other he believed things would work out.

One day in the summer of 1954, two of his college friends, Chung Byung Uk and Lee He Won, suggested that they attend the Ecumenical International Church near Duksoo Palace in Seoul. It would be a new experience where they would hear English spoken in a religious setting.

The Ecumenical service and sermon were conducted and delivered by the U.S. Army Chaplain. At the end of the service, the Chaplain stood at the door of the Church greeting the attendees. One by one, people shook hands with the Chaplain, a Colonel, and exchanged a few words of greetings.

"I enjoyed your sermon, Sir," said Andrew as his turn came.

The Colonel's eyes lit up with surprise. "You speak good English."

"Thank you, Sir."

"I mean it! Are you a student? Where? At Seoul National University? What are you doing this afternoon?"

"Nothing, Sir."

"Do you know where the 8th Army Headquarters is in Yongsan? I would like for you to visit me this afternoon, if you can."

"Thank you Sir, I would be happy to visit you, but I can't get past the gate."

"Just come to the gate and ask the Military Policeman or M.P. to call Colonel Sidney Crumpton. The M.P. should then bring you to my office without any difficulty. "

Surprised by the encounter and invitation, Andrew's friends urged him to keep his promise to visit the Chaplain, certain that an offer for a part-time job might follow.

So later that afternoon, Andrew appeared at the gate of the 8th Army Headquarters in Seoul and asked the M.P. for Colonel Sidney Crumpton. Following a call to the Colonel, he was promptly taken by jeep to Colonel Crumpton's Office in one of the many tents in the area.

After the usual greetings, the Colonel launched in by asking about Andrew's family and educational history.

He began by telling the Colonel that his Father was a physician and that he had lost both parents in the war, completely avoiding the traumatic details. He then talked about completing high school and his admission to Seoul National University in pre-medicine.

The Colonel listened politely, offered Andrew his first taste of Coca Cola, showed him the location of the various units of the 8th Army Headquarters and so forth for about a half hour, all the while nodding his head whenever Andrew responded to his leading questions.

Then rather suddenly, he turned, looked directly at the young man and asked, "Would you like to study in America?"

Andrew was taken aback by the query, but answered, "Yes, but I cannot because I cannot afford it."

"What if you had a full scholarship?"

"Yes of course, if I had a full scholarship, I would like to study medicine in America."

"That could be arranged, we'll see to that," said the Colonel, to Andrew's great surprise.

A few minutes later, the Colonel called for the driver of the jeep to return the visitor to the tram stop for his return home with the parting promise that he would get in touch with him again, before too long.

The experience was quite unusual for Andrew, especially coming on the heels of all the upheavals in his life and the stresses of life in the immediate postwar period. To say the least, it promised more than he had ever imagined possible. It seemed to him to be another sign of hope from the Almighty.

A few days later, he was summoned to report to Professor Chun, of the English Department at Seoul National University, who was also the Registrar.

Entering the office, Andrew noticed Professor Chun was wearing a quizzical look, as if he knew something he wished he didn't.

"Do you know Chaplain Crumpton?" he asked after the usual greetings were completed.

Andrew acknowledged that he did, having only met him a week before, when he was asked to visit him at his office at the U.S. 8th Army Base in Seoul, he explained.

"The Colonel wants me to tell you that if you want to go to America, you would be given a full scholarship. Of course, you must obtain your Grandfather's permission, first," he added, seemingly at odds with the content of his message, perhaps wishing Tiger's Grandfather might object.

Undoubtedly, he was happy for Andrew on the one hand, but on the other, he was disappointed at the prospect of losing one of his most promising students for studies abroad.

Andrew explained about his Grandfather, that he was bedridden as a result of a recent stroke. However, he would inform him and determine whether he approved or not of his acceptance of an education in medicine in the U.S. before taking the scholarship, he promised the Registrar.

As the visit drew to a close, Professor Chun asked Andrew if he had ever read a book of a particular title, where a boy is in a field of dreams of good things happening to him. Well, he would tell of an updated story with a similar content, he promised.

"I was visited by Colonel Crumpton, who was recently visited by a student, namely you. The Colonel wanted to know who you were and if we had any crackerjack students worthy of a full scholarship to Wofford College in South Carolina in the U.S. I told him that you were the top dog at school and he virtually jumped up and down!" said Professor Chun.

From the Professor's look of projected delight and the wide smile on Andrew's face, it was not clear who the dreamer was, Andrew, the Professor, or Colonel Crumpton.

Overjoyed to hear this offer, Andrew could hardly contain himself.

Of course his Grandfather approved, gesturing as best as he could from his bed to convey his happiness that his Grandson would be studying abroad on a scholarship. Having converted to Catholicism, he even appeared to bless Andrew with movements that he made with his right hand.   -

Unawares, Andrew still had a hierarchy of hurdles to overcome. It would take him between 8-9 months to obtain a visa to enter the U.S. There was the Korean Foreign Minister's Office where a passport application had to be filled out; papers had to be filed with the Korean Department of Defense to be granted an exemption from the draft; and the American Consulate Office had other papers to be filled and filed where he was treated as at no other time in his life. It was not simply the remoteness of the bureaucratic personality that he noticed, but more like the expression of racial bias he had experienced from a few Japanese soldiers before their defeat.

A final roadblock with the American Consulate's Office was to procure an acceptable required Affidavit of Support from an American. Who would be able to provide this, considering that none of Andrew's relatives could afford to do so and none was an American?

A compromise was finally reached between the Governments of Korea and the U.S., where Wofford College guaranteed fare to the U.S. and the scholarship, while his Grandfather's brother, who had been educated in Germany and was a Korean diplomat, guaranteed financial support and Andrew's fare back to Korea.

With each of these transactions, he had to draft letters by himself for the signatories to sign. While his verbal skills in English were satisfactory, his writing was less well advanced especially for such official and legal documents, such that each letter became a writing ordeal, requiring hours apiece.

Furthermore, each letter needed to be posted via airmail to Wofford College at some expense to him, taxing his already meager miscellaneous fund, especially with runaway inflation in Korea. Finally, everything was approved and Andrew was ready to depart for "medical school" in the U.S.

At that time, Andrew was not aware that the medical education system in Korea differed significantly from that in the U.S. Whereas, admission to a college in medicine meant a six-year period of study at the same college after which the M.D. degree was awarded in Korea, in the U.S. the study of medicine was accomplished through two separate steps.

First, one was admitted to a college for a baccalaureate degree after which a separate application had to be made for medical school for another four years of study.

Unaware of the difference, he believed he was admitted for study towards a medical degree by his acceptance to Wofford College.

Meanwhile, his elder sister, Ok Im was getting of an age where marriage had to be considered. By custom, suitable arrangements are made by the parents of the bride through the intercession of intermediaries, either related or professional, the so-called marriage brokers. During the long process of gaining a visa to study in the U.S., arrangements were also being made for Ok Im to be married through the intercession of his relatives.

Chung Byung Uk, the friend with whose family he had lived in Pusan while attending Kyonggi High School during the war, had a relative working for a Chinese business firm in Seoul, who expressed interest in marrying her. Formal permission was obtained from Uncle Choi Han Woong, the pediatrician, and the marriage took place several months before Andrew was scheduled to depart for the U.S.

Now it would be his younger sister, Duk Im, who would supervise the younger siblings and manage the household. She would be entering college and was mature enough to manage everything for the rest of his siblings, he reassured himself. A few months of practice ensured Andrew of her ability to wisely oversee the family's needs in his absence.

CHAPTER 8: TIGER GOES WEST

On April 13, 1955, family and friends came to bid Andrew goodbye at the old civilian airport in Seoul, located on Yoi-do Island surrounded by the waters of the Han River.

Andrew had a single suitcase holding his personal belongings, a one-way ticket to Spartanburg, South Carolina via Wake Island, Honolulu, Los Angeles, Dallas, and Atlanta and five hundred U.S. dollars in his wallet.

To make his transition to the West more tolerable, he was given a jar of kochu-jang, a spicy hot, garlic-flavored soybean sauce, to use to blank out any foreign, bland, or undesirable taste in the unfamiliar foods he would undoubtedly encounter, the giver had told him.

So armed, he boarded the propeller plane and waved goodbye to his family, friends, and homeland.

Flying was a novel experience for him. Before the end of World War II, he had traveled at least twice a year by train to the north to spend several weeks with his paternal

Grandfather at Iwon, now in North Korea. The journey by train was long and he always traveled with a lacquered wooden box tied within a colorful square of cloth containing a full meal to eat en route.

At the end of the journey, he was met by one or another family member and taken by oxen driven cart to a large farmhouse where he was treated to the best of everything by a doting Grandfather who had selected the name "Ho" or Tiger for his eldest son's first-born son.

It was unusual to use a single word or syllable for a name, but the Grandfather had no doubt that his first Grandson bearing the surname of Kang would be called "Ho" for Tiger with no other nominal feature necessary. At home in Seoul, the elders called him In-sohn, or a Tiger of a Grandson while his classmates called him Ho-rang, the usual word for a tiger in ordinary reference to the four-footed animal. Officially, he was Kang Ho in South Korea, but was Andrew Ho Kang on his visa to the U.S., and would continue to be Andrew Ho Kang, thenceforth.

Strapped in his seat on the airplane, Tiger, Ho, In-sohn, Ho-rang, and Andrew, all bundled together in one person peered out of the window and watched his beloved country gradually receding away from his field of vision.

It was certainly a rugged land with mountains and hills occupying the majority of the territory, now divided into two irreconcilable halves, sticking out into the seas as a peninsula off the eastern edge of the huge continent of Asia. The southern half was now struggling to emerge with a viable, democratic form of government. It was sandwiched between China and Japan with Manchuria and Russia to the north. Each of these countries had made aggressive attempts to subjugate the rabbit-shaped, mountainous country called at various times, the Land of the Morning Calm, the Hermit Kingdom, Chosun, and Korea.

At least, a portion of the country was free and one day, the entire country would be united and free, he almost prayed.

He was leaving his family behind knowing the financial arrangements he had coped with would continue to support them despite his absence. In fact, the small amount of money he had been earning by tutoring other students at night would be replaced by the savings arising from a reduction in the family's total expenses brought on by his absence, he reasoned.

Pondering these practical issues, he was soon lulled into sleep by the droning sounds of the propeller driven airplane. The brief stop at Wake Island to refuel hardly woke him.

His flight to the various portals of entry in the U.S. was uneventful except for the stop in Honolulu. The plane had landed and everyone was exiting. The scheduled flight from Honolulu to Los Angeles was several hours away and Andrew thought he might deplane and look around, also.

Once in the airport itself, he turned to do just that, looking around, when suddenly the paper sack in which the kochujang bottle was held slipped and smashed on the hard, concrete floor.

The shattering glass shards broke the paper sack, spilling the contents like ooze on the floor. Immediately, a pungent odor of fully fermented soybean paste generously flavored with garlic filled the air.

Jolted by the abruptness of the accident and a bit embarrassed, Andrew bit his lower lip and then muttered in a long drawn out whisper, "Ssshhett!" Whatever English he had learned from the American troops in Korea was certainly put to good use, he thought. At least, it sounded just right!

Passengers and visitors around him wrinkled their noses because of the odor, quickly side-stepping the area.

Tempted to walk away to leave the cleaning to the housekeeping staff, Andrew nearly walked off. Just as luck would have it, before him, he spied a newspaper rack. Without another second's thought, he walked toward it with deliberate steps, stuck in some change he had obtained before the trip, retrieved a paper, returned to the spillage site and immediately scooped up the debris and remnants. He walked to the nearest trash bin and dumped the mess with deliberate motions, finally brushing his hands together to rid himself of a few fragments of sticky paper.

Much relieved, he quickly sought a place to wash up. Glad to be rid of the package, which he would otherwise have had to lug all the way to Spartanburg, South Carolina, he nevertheless wondered if he hadn't lost something precious.

On the final leg of his long journey from Atlanta to Spartanburg, Andrew peered out of the airplane window as before. His thoughts returned to the incredible series of events following that Sunday five years before when he heard the distant thud, thud heralding the beginning of unbelievable events and great upheavals in his life and the world about him.

He solemnly resolved to complete his education with the highest honors possible for someone with his language and financial handicaps and then to return to Korea to help the rest of his family and his own beloved country.

Would the North and South ever unite, he wondered to himself? It was more likely that the North would reattempt a takeover of the South, he said to himself raising the specter of a continuing danger long into the future.

He proceeded logically to review whether all contingencies were adequately provided for his siblings in Korea and to consider his own priorities.

Somewhere, somehow after he completed his studies, he would have to find his Father, or at least learn of his fate. As for his Mother, he short circuited recalling the events surrounding his search for her, but reassured himself that she would very likely have approved of his choice to study medicine in the U.S.

His younger siblings would complete their education under the guidance of Uncle Han Woong Choi and others of his extended family. His sister OK Im's marriage had been finalized. Routine matters of managing the household would continue under the supervision of the sister just below him, Duk Im, who was smart as a whip and very competent. His other sisters, Bok Im and Kyung Im, were young teenagers now, certainly able to contribute to the running of the household. His younger brother, Pyo (Leopard), was an excellent student, though often uncomfortably quiet and withdrawn, but would pose no challenge to his sisters. There should be no need to worry about his siblings, he rationalized, bringing closure to various aspects that had burdened him previously.

Now he would focus on the work that lay ahead of him.

Photos

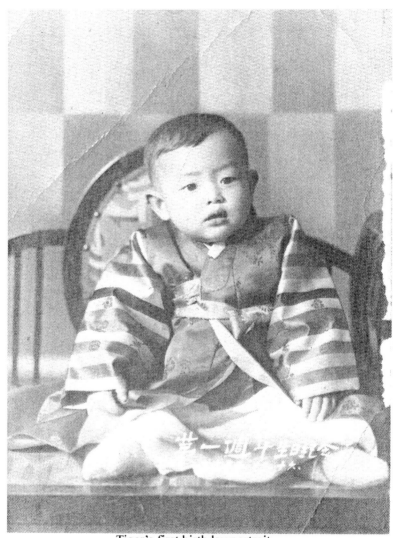

Tiger's first birthday portrait.

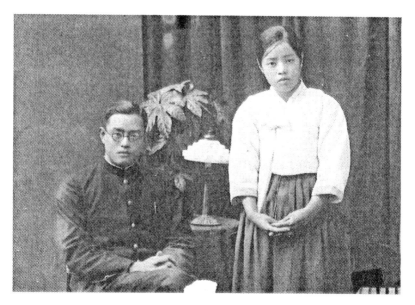

Tiger's Parents.

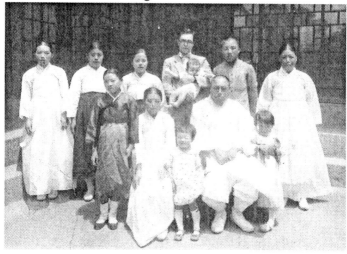

Paternal Grandparents' family in Iwon, Korea
[Grandparents, seated. Center, back row, Tiger's Mother and Father
(holding Tiger as infant)]

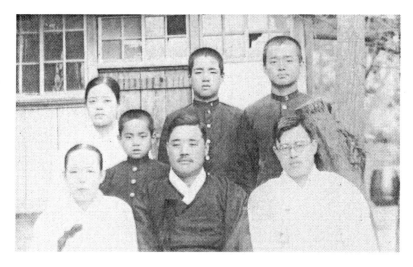

Maternal Grandparents' family in Seoul, Korea
[Seated: Grandmother, Grandfather (Choi Nam Sun), and Tiger's
Father. Standing, Tiger's Mother, an Uncle, Uncle Choi Han Woong,
and another Uncle]

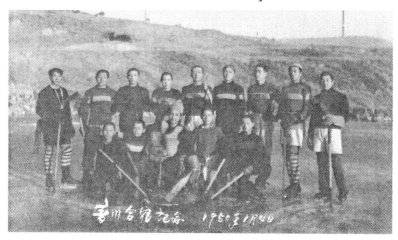

Kyonggi School hockey team, 1950.
[Tiger, kneeling, second from left]

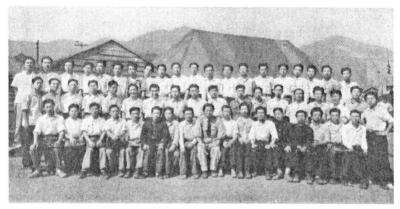

Kyonggi High School Class after evacuation to Pusan
[Tiger, back row, sixth from the right]

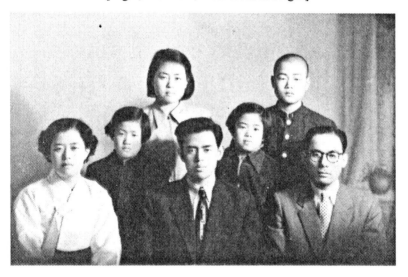

Last portrait with siblings before Tiger's departure for the U.S.
[Seated, first row: Elder sister, Ok Im, Andrew (Tiger), Ok Im's husband,
Mr. Song. Standing, second row: Kyung Im (youngest sister), Bok Im
(3rd sister). Top row: Duk Im (2nd sister), brother Pyo]

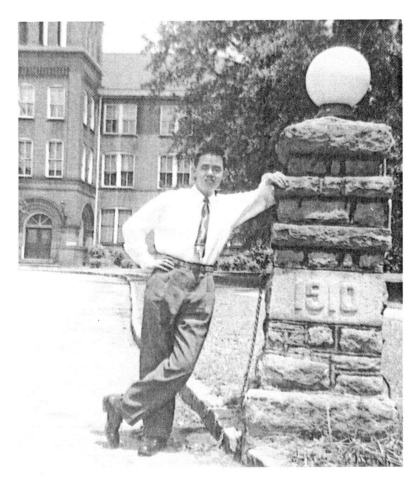

Andrew at college in Spartanburg, S.C.

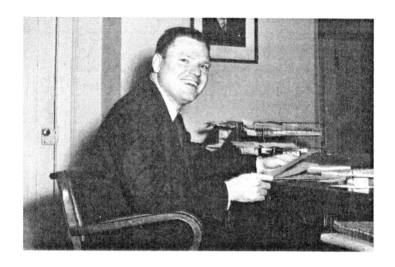

Mr. Frank Logan, Dean of Students, Wofford College, Spartanburg, S.C.

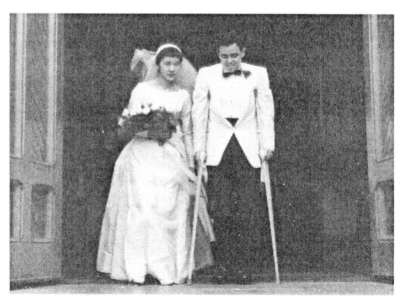

After the wedding, September 6, 1958.

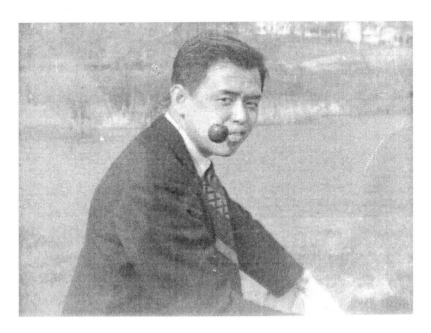

Andrew at Fenway

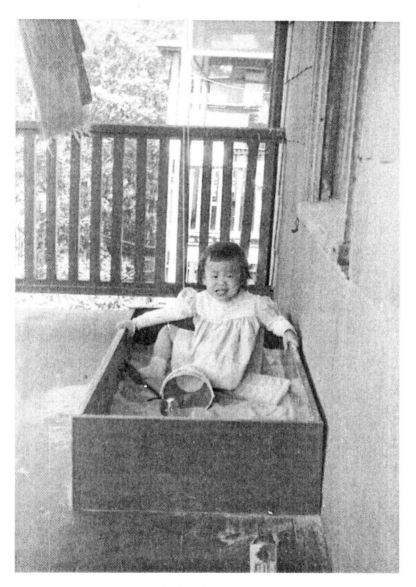

Cynthia enjoying first piece of carpentry

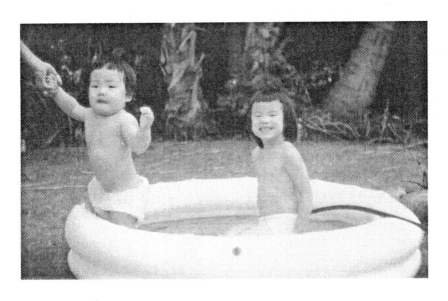

Edith and Cynthia in Hawaii

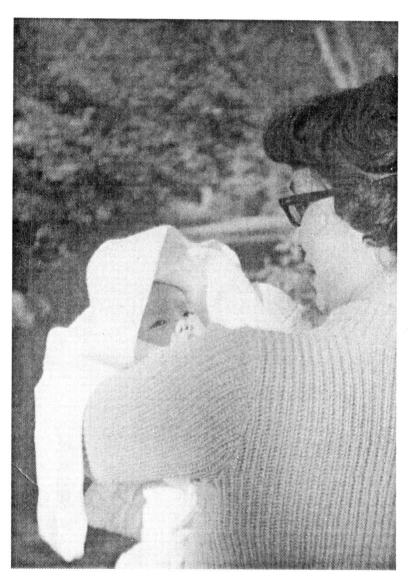

Audrey, peering at her Mother.

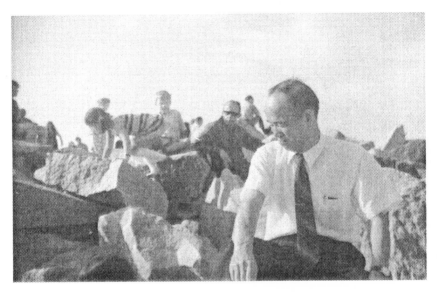

Uncle Choi Han Woong during visit, Rockport, MA.
[Edith climbing on rocks in striped dress]

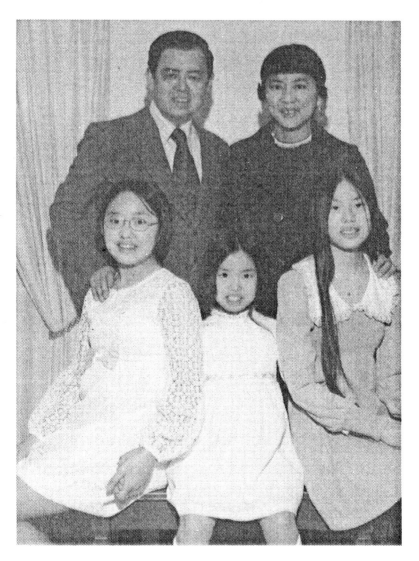

After the family's move to Memphis, TN.
[Seated L-R: daughters, Edith, Audrey and Cynthia]

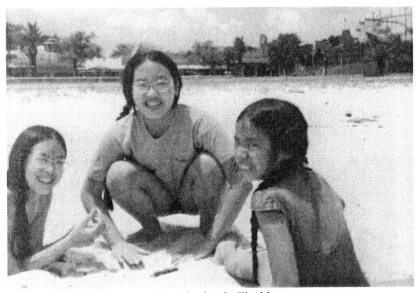

Vacationing in Florida.
[Daughters, L-R: Cynthia, Edith, and Audrey]

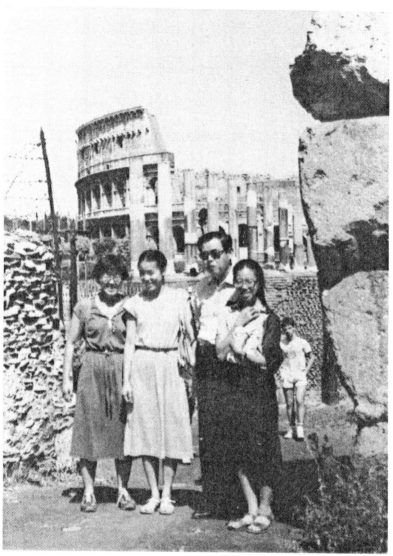

2nd visit to Rome with daughters, Coloseum.

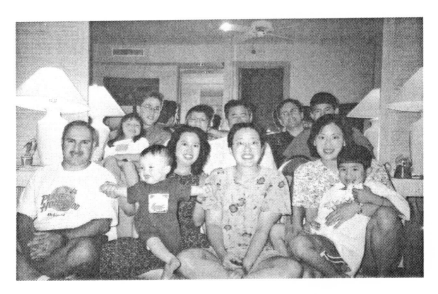

Extended Family at Captiva, Florida.
[Including 3 sons-in-law and four grandchildren]

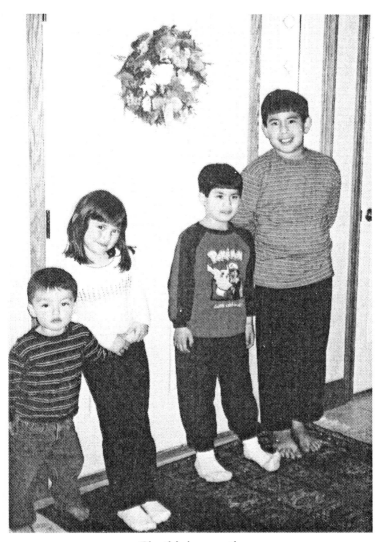

The third generation.
[Grandchildren from L-R: Jonathan Tae In David, Caitlin Mi
Sun David, Matthew Joseph Rotondo, and Jeffrey Andrew Rotondo]

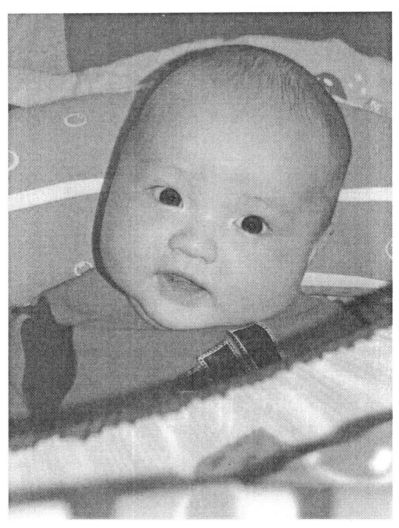

The Fifth grandchild: Nicholas Yong In Tesauro arrived on August 8, 2005 to Audrey and Tom Tesauro

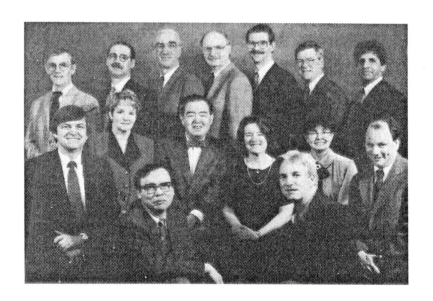

The Connective Tissue Research Laboratory in 1994
[Front row, L->R: Dr. Tom Chiang, Dr. Bill Watson; middle row: Dr. John Stuart, Dr. Karen Hasty, Dr. Andrew Kang, Dr. Linda Myers, Dr. Gloria Higgins, Dr. David Brand; Back row: Dr. Jerry Seyer, Dr. Carlo Mainardi, Dr. Arnold Postlethwaite, Dr. Mike Cremer, Dr. Ed Rosloniec, Dr. Les Ballou, and Dr. Raj Raghow]

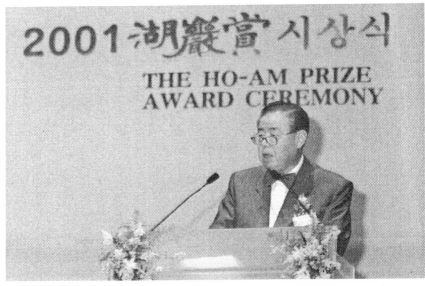

Dr. Andrew Ho Kang delivering a speech on receipt of the Ho-Am Prize in Medicine from the Ho-Am Foundation of Korea.

CHAPTER 9: WOFFORD COLLEGE AND SPARTANBURG, S.C.

It was the morning of the 15th of April in 1955 when the plane landed at Spartanburg, South Carolina. Mr. Frank Logan, the Registrar at Wofford College in Spartanburg, S.C., had written earlier that he would meet Andrew at the airport. The plane was small, and so was the airport. It would be easy to locate each other, Andrew figured.

Everyone deplaned.

No one appeared to be waiting for him, so he followed the crowd towards the baggage area. Midway there, a man with a felt hat hurried toward him.

"Are you Andrew Kang? I'm Frank Logan, the Registrar," he said as he stretched out his hand.

They picked up the single suitcase at the luggage area and proceeded to Mr. Logan's Studebaker for the short ride to the campus, all the while engaging in conversation.

"Gosh, you speak good English," Mr. Logan said.

This seemed strange to Andrew, who nevertheless thanked him politely.

Reaching the dormitory, Mr. Logan left him to settle down and asked him to come by his office the next morning in a nearby building, which he pointed out.

Andrew located his assigned dormitory room, unpacked, and found his way around, meeting others briefly as most were busy studying.

Everything was new and different and he seemed to be the only Asian around. Everyone else was Caucasoid. Most were taller and much broader than he was, sporting brown or blonde hair with very light skin, and a few had freckled flecks of darker color scattered about their cheeks and noses. Several had red hair, a very unusual color to him.

The men of the Allied Forces in Taegu and Seoul had their hair shorn off in a uniform sort of way and no one noticed whether one was a blonde or brunette. Now he saw hair of various lengths and colors on everyone around him.

All the while, others in the dormitory looked with surprise to find an Asian, who was almost as tall as they were with wavy, black hair and a wide personable, somewhat toothy smile, who promptly responded to their greetings with his own "Hi, how are you?"

Finally, after a large evening meal at the dormitory dining hall in the company of a few newly found friends, Andrew fell asleep, exhausted after a long, long journey that ended with his introduction to an entirely new way of life amongst the friendliest cadre of young men he could have imagined.

The next morning, he made it to Mr. Logan's office before 10 a.m. After their greeting and hand shaking, Mr. Logan ushered Andrew into the Conference Room.

There he picked out a book from one of the shelves bordering the room and turned the book over to Andrew, asking him to read what was printed on a randomly selected page.

Andrew obliged after which Mr. Logan asked him if he understood what he had read.

"I think so," Andrew replied, proceeding to explain what it was that he had just read.

Mr. Logan had a pensive look about him before he explained that it was only a month away from final examinations. He suggested that it might be better if Andrew audited the courses and not bother with the final examinations.

Accordingly, he proceeded to the first of his classes, Algebra, taught by Mr. Ken Coates who had already been informed of the new student from Korea.

Mr. Coates kindly introduced the newly arrived student to the class, which numbered about a dozen students.

"Oh, bad luck, Mr. Kang, today is the day for a pop test. You could leave or take the test, whatever you wish to do," he offered.

Of course, Andrew took the test. The test questions were rather easy for him, except that he was not certain about the Korean equivalent of a square as opposed to a rectangle, critical to the solution of one of the problems in the test. Nonetheless, he completed the test in 10 minutes, feeling confident that he had done well.

At the next meeting of the class two days later, Mr. Coates announced to the class that whereas Mr. Kang had not taken the course, he had missed only one problem, making a 75, higher than many who had taken the course.

Andrew was mortified and heard nothing else the rest of the hour. After class, he approached the teacher. "Sir, I have never made a 75 in any test before, and I am ashamed," he said.

He continued, explaining that he did not know the Korean equivalent of a square as opposed to a rectangle, the reason for missing the problem. He had not brought either of the two dictionaries to class that he needed, the Korean/English and the English/Korean dictionaries, he said with considerable chagrin and embarrassment.

Mr. Coates believed him and saw that Andrew had a good grasp of Algebra except for the vocabulary matter, which he would conquer in time. After a slight pause during which he slowly nodded his head as though he understood more than was being said, he suggested that they meet with the Chairman of the Mathematics Department.

After a brief explanation by Mr. Coates, the Chairman, Mr. Hill, suggested that Andrew audit Calculus 102 with the view that if he passed the final examination, only four weeks away, credit would be given to him for both Algebra and Calculus.

As it was, Calculus 102 was taught by Mr. Hill himself. Andrew sat up front in the first row, in order to lip read as well as listen to maximize his understanding of each lecture.

After a statement or explanation, Mr. Hill would invariably turn to him and ask, "Did you understand that, Mr. Kang?"

Each time, Andrew answered, "Yes, Sir."

After the nth time, he replied raising the decibel of his voice just a trifle but noticeable bit, "Of course, Sir!"

At this polite but strong response, the whole class broke out in laughter.

There followed a slight, somewhat uncomfortable pause. Then, Mr. Hill erased everything off the board and slowly jotted down another, completely different problem.

He slowly turned around and addressed the whole class, asking whether anyone had a solution or might attempt to solve the problem. "Anyone?" he asked, looking at the entire class from right to left and back to right.

In the absence of a response, he turned to Andrew seated directly in front of him and asked him, "Mr. Kang, would you mind solving this problem?"

"Of course, Sir," came the cock-sure answer. However, Andrew was struck by a momentary memory lapse of the formula necessary to solve the problem.

He quickly flipped the textbook on his desk toward the Appendices in the back. Incredibly, he had reached the very page with the formula needed to solve the problem. With an instantaneous glance, the formula reregistered in his mind.

He strode confidently toward the board, completing the calculations in his head, and chalked the answer on the board without a pause, but with a bit of flourish.

"Would you mind explaining how you arrived at the answer, Mr. Kang?" asked Mr. Hill withholding his amusement at the bit of comical drama he witnessed being acted out in his ordinarily dour class.

"Me no speak good English, but—," said Andrew, with tongue in cheek.

Turning around to the board with deliberate steps, he proceeded to jot the several logical mathematical sequences that would lead the class to the correct answer.

Everyone marveled at his performance, as did Mr. Hill. At the end of class, Mr. Hill asked him to stay behind for a few minutes.

"You obviously have taken Calculus before," Mr. Hill began.

Andrew told him that he had calculus-like courses several years before in high school, but not a formal course called Calculus at Seoul National University. Not knowing the entire elements included in Calculus 102 and having forgotten many of the formulas he had learned in high school, he was not sure that he would qualify as having had a college course equivalent to the one Mr. Hill was teaching at Wofford.

After a moment of thought, Mr. Hill informed him that an intermediate test was to be given in a week. If he passed the examination, he would be given credit for Algebra and the course work in Calculus up to the present time. "That's a promise," Mr. Hill offered.

Andrew took the examination and, of course, passed with a perfect score. He was given credit for Algebra and was registered in Calculus, as promised.

During the same period, Andrew also appeared to be doing well in Biology taught by Mr. Leonard. After one of Mr. Leonard's lectures, a group of students had gathered, discussing what they believed Mr. Leonard had covered in the lecture. Andrew was there and disagreed with the interpretation given by one of the members of the group.

Mr. Leonard, the instructor was passing by, when he stopped and tapped Andrew aside. He asked Andrew whether he had any questions noting the dubious look Andrew had on his face.

Andrew thought Mr. Leonard was asking about the student's interpretation of the lecture content.

"I think it's a bunch of bull!" came the quick response.

Quietly aghast, Mr. Leonard suggested, "Mr. Kang, you probably don't understand what you just said!"

He proceeded to explain the social inappropriateness of Andrew's response and then clarified the lecture subject, which, of course, matched Andrew's understanding.

Somewhat taken aback, Andrew apologized for his inappropriate verbal response. He took Mr. Leonard's advice to heart and thenceforth was a bit more careful in his choice of vernacular terms, at least in the presence of his teachers.

Over the coming months and years, Mr. Leonard befriended the young man from Korea, who continued to learn and follow his advice as given from time to time, whenever indicated.

Other instructors in Chemistry, Physics, and German soon came to recognize that Andrew had knowledge ordinarily acquired after nearly two semesters of instruction in their courses, despite the fact that he had only just arrived less than three weeks before.

One day several weeks after Andrew had been at Wofford, Mr. Logan, the Registrar, asked Andrew to his office. He said that he had excellent reports of Andrew's work from every instructor. Final examinations were looming just ahead and every instructor was willing to allow him to take the finals and would provide credit for the full course, if he passed.

Andrew agreed to prepare for the examinations, not realizing that he was about to embark on one of the greatest challenges of his young life as a student. He had studied many of the concepts and elements in these courses several years before in high school in Korea as well as during the year at Seoul National University. However, here everything would be in English, requiring frequent use of the dictionaries and his translating back and forth between the two languages with every unfamiliar word. And, such words were present in nearly every paragraph he encountered.

Because of his language handicap, he had to spend much precious time rifling through both word aid books, the Korean/American and the American/Korean Dictionaries. Pace in covering the entire subject areas of each of the courses was thereby slow and painful. Every evening, he stayed awake until way past midnight to prepare for the exams.

In addition, it was already hot in South Carolina and air conditioning was not available. Moreover, he could not work with the window open because of the noisiness outside the dormitory. Somehow or other, he managed to persevere and concentrate, wiping off beads of sweat off his forehead and face with his handkerchief and drinking lots of water.

He was also not used to objective examinations, having had to write out passages during tests for most of his courses in Korea. A bit anxious about his overall performance on these tests, he was pleasantly surprised to learn a few days later that he had passed with highly respectable grades.

As expected, Mr. Logan was also quite pleased. After less than six weeks at the college, he was given credit for a whole year's work for each of the courses that he had originally registered only to audit.

Thus, the college year ended. Andrew moved to the local YMCA on Main Street in Spartanburg for several days until summer courses would begin at Wofford College. Mr. Logan had arranged for this transition as well as for a temporary job typing labels for fifty cents an hour.

It was during this time when he learned of the circumstances that led to his selection for the scholarship at

Wofford by Chaplain Crumpton, the 8th Army Chaplain in Seoul, Korea, from Mr. Logan.

Apparently, the local Rotary Club in Spartanburg had taken upon itself to sponsor a student from Korea in honor of Wofford's Centennial Celebration. Many members had served in the Korean War, returning with vivid memories of the appalling tragedies that the civilians had faced and wanting to contribute something towards the emerging democracy of Korea.

A student named Kim, who was to have entered Seoul National University, was selected to receive the honor, a full scholarship to Wofford College. Kim arrived at Wofford a year before, but had great difficulty adjusting to the work and the college community. He frequently cut classes, complained of being terribly homesick, and did poorly in his courses, seemingly unable to find a friend.

The Administrators at Wofford were anxious to fulfill their objective, namely to educate a young man from the previously war-torn Korea. They persuaded the Rotary Club to allow them to seek another candidate through Colonel Crumpton, who was then serving as a Chaplain in the 8th Army located in Seoul. They expected that Kim might adjust in the company of another student of Korean ancestry.

Accordingly, the Chaplain had been on the lookout for just such a student when Andrew appeared and spoke up so confidently at the conclusion of the Ecumenical Service. Crumpton had informed them that he had identified a socially friendly, English speaking student who turned out to be the top student in the Freshman Class at Seoul National University.

However, before Andrew's arrival, the unhappy student Kim had returned to Korea and dropped all further contact with Wofford College.

Nevertheless, the Rotary Club agreed to go through with Andrew's scholarship offer. Of course, everyone waited with considerable anxiety to see how the second student would do, not only in adjusting to America, Spartanburg, South Carolina, and to Wofford and campus life, but also to separation from his homeland and culture.

Much to their delight, "Andrew had turned out to be a Tiger, true to form, living up to his Korean name of Ho," Mr. Logan said, who had learned that Ho stood for Tiger.

Just before summer courses began, Andrew returned to the college dormitory. Two courses were selected, the Old Testament and Philosophy, both requiring much reading. The dictionaries he had brought with him from Korea were heavily utilized.

Now, he also learned how much hotter the heat of summer in South Carolina could be, hardly bearable even after the sun had gone down. Were it not for the electric fan that he bought, he might not have survived that summer of hard work.

About this time, he learned for the first time that entry to medical school in the U.S. required two separate processes, unlike Korea. Following completion of undergraduate work, another application had to be made for graduate studies in medicine, where competition was fierce for a limited number of spaces.

Wofford offered a baccalaureate degree in a number of areas, but did not have a graduate school, and was not linked to a medical college. Individual states with state sponsored medical schools accepted their own residents, who had to be citizens of the U.S. Some state medical schools would accept a selected number of residents of adjoining states, who also had to be U.S. citizens. Private medical schools would consider candidates without preference as to their residency or citizenship, provided they were academically suitable. Furthermore, tuition costs at private medical schools were much, much higher than at state schools.

Considering these factors, there was little else that Andrew could do but to study as hard as possible in order to win a scholarship to a private medical school. Each day, he studied until 5 p.m., took a half hour off to eat his supper and promptly continued studying until midnight. This formula worked nicely and he passed all of the courses he took with flying colors.

With the close of the summer session, Andrew moved to a small apartment attached to the garage of the home of a friend of Mr. Logan's until classes at Wofford would resume in the fall. He was also paid to baby sit for the Logans. Over the course of time, friendship between the Logans and Andrew grew strong. In fact, they seemed to have become Andrew's surrogate parents.

In September, he was back in the dormitory and registered for Organic Chemistry, Comparative Anatomy, English Literature, History and Political Science. There was not a doubt anymore about his learning abilities and he disappointed no one.

Andrew had begun attending the local Episcopal Church upon his initial arrival in Spartanburg, S.C. and before long was befriended by Dr. and Mrs. George Johnson, both of whom were extremely active church members.

Once, he was invited to the Johnsons' home for "dinner" on a Sunday, which he accepted along with another invitation from yet another family for lunch the same day. He showed up for lunch with the other family, which he enjoyed very much. Later, when he arrived for "dinner" at the Johnsons, he learned that "Sunday dinner" was actually meant for lunch, the largest meal on Sunday in the South. He learned that he had been missed at Sunday dinner by the Johnsons, who, nevertheless, invited him in for the evening meal.

Despite this faux pas, he was subsequently invited again for an evening dinner along with his roommate, George Sally.

Prior to appearing at the Johnsons, Andrew had expressed some concern to his roommate about his inability to properly use the several table utensils that would be set before him at the Johnsons.

For a crash lesson in western etiquette, his roommate advised him to simply watch him as they worked through the meal. And, indeed, George Sally succeeded in guiding him through the rudiments of western table grace rather smoothly.

The Johnsons befriended Andrew, inviting him back for meals quite frequently, and also inviting him to spend part of the Christmas holidays and a few weeks in the summers with them.

In time, Mr. Logan became the Dean of Students. Whether through Mr. Logan's aegis or not, somehow or other, word got out to others in the community of Andrew's social and linguistic appeal and he was invited to speak at the local Rotary Club as well as at Youth Meetings at the Episcopal and other local churches. (Many years later, Andrew learned from an administrator at Harvard Medical School that Mr. Logan's letters about Andrew were such heartfelt ones that they could wring blood out of a turnip.)

During his second full year at Wofford, he began applying to medical school. Most of his pre-medicine classmates were applying to the University of South Carolina. Andrew's application to the state supported University of South Carolina School of Medicine was refused on the basis of his non-citizenship. Scouring through the medical catalogues at the school library for a listing of private medical schools, he selected Jefferson, Harvard, Duke, Emory, Tulane and Baylor University Medical Schools for application. With each application, he notified the school of his need for a full scholarship.

Duke University was prompt in its reply—no full scholarship was offered to a freshman, and his application would not be considered further unless the condition for a scholarship was removed, which of course he could not.

Tulane was the first school that responded positively, requiring that Andrew come to New Orleans, Louisiana for an interview.

He did just that, traveling by bus. He was accepted shortly thereafter with the condition that he forward a deposit of fifty dollars to hold his spot. However, no full scholarship had been offered and Andrew consulted Mr. Logan about the matter.

"Take it first, and then we can explore the possibility of financing your education later," Mr. Logan wisely advised him.

Jefferson Medical School accepted Andrew's application without an interview, offered no scholarship, and requested a deposit of twenty-five dollars.

Baylor stated they had a policy about not awarding scholarships to freshmen, but that they were willing to work with the Rotary Club for a scholarship for the-01 year. They required an interview, however. Mr. Logan had already written to each school and learned that Baylor was willing to pay for Andrew's travel to Dallas, Texas for the interview.

Just about the same time, Harvard notified Andrew that his interview with them could be accomplished through Dr. Lloyd Smith in Easley, South Carolina. However, as it turned out, Dr. Smith was no longer living in Easley, South Carolina, having more recently moved to Boston, Massachusetts.

Shortly thereafter, Harvard sent the name of another alumnus who would interview him, Dr. William Pitts of Charlotte, North Carolina. It was kind Mr. Logan who drove Andrew to the interview, some 70 miles north of Spartanburg, S.C.

Dr. Pitts was a surgeon who interviewed Andrew all dressed in his surgical gown complete with headgear.

At the end of the interview, Mr. Logan introduced himself. "I'm the Dean of Students at Wofford College, can I have a talk with you?" he asked.

They talked behind closed doors for about a half hour after which both reappeared and everyone parted after the usual niceties.

It wasn't until a few days later when Mr. Logan called Andrew into his office that Andrew could guess about what had been said during their brief conference behind closed doors. Dr. Pitts had sent a check for a hundred dollars for Andrew's use.

Several days later, a telephone call arrived at the dormitory for Andrew. It was a Western Union clerk, who read the telegram just received. "Congratulations, you are accepted to Harvard Medical School. Please reply."

He was glad but disappointed at the same time because of the absence of any mention of a scholarship. With help from his roommate George Sally, he wrote back to Harvard stating that he needed a scholarship in order to accept admission to Harvard.

The response from Harvard was prompt: scholarships were not awarded until the class was fully constituted. Furthermore, once admitted, no student had ever had to leave because of financial insufficiency, the letter stated.

He therefore accepted admission to Harvard Medical School, fully trusting that financial support would be forthcoming, somehow or other. His experiences with Americans to date assured him that they kept their word.

The Baylor interview was cancelled. He wrote to Tulane Medical College, asking for a refund of the fifty dollar deposit. A polite letter returned indicating that it was not their usual policy to refund a deposit, but they did enclose a check for fifty dollars.

He had mentioned these developments to Dr. George Johnson, who was a Jefferson Medical School graduate. Not long after, a check for the amount of the deposit was also returned to Andrew from Jefferson Medical School, to Andrew's surprise and delight.

Eventually, official notice did arrive from Harvard advising him of full financial support for the duration of his medical education at Harvard, provided his work was satisfactory. The burden he had shouldered upon first learning that the scholarship to Wofford College did not include support for his medical education, was finally lifted.

By Christmas of 1956, plans for the future seemed to be taking shape rather well. To add to his good fortune, Mrs. George Johnson, the good doctor's wife, gathered her companions at the Women's Club of the Episcopal Church to mount a "Get Andrew Ready for Medical School Drive."

They collected clothes suitable for a doctor, including a brown suit with a vest, yes, a matching vest, a pair of leather shoes, a heavy herring-bone coat for the colder New England weather complete with a removable lining, shirts and trousers to wear to class as well as church, ties of various colors to match his clothes, sweaters, and even T-shirts, undies and socks.

He was escorted to a men's clothier for a special gray suit to be tailored under Mrs. Johnson's keen discriminating eye. In addition, a fund was established by the Women's Club to raise money for Andrew's personal use as a medical student.

There was a burgeoning of goodwill and kindness from the people of the Episcopal Church of Spartanburg, South Carolina and Wofford College, all lavished upon the young man from Seoul, Korea. To physically accommodate the gifts he had received, a footlocker had to be purchased.

In June of 1957, he graduated from Wofford College, receiving his B.S. degree in Biology Summa Cum Laude and was elected to Phi Beta Kappa. Mr. Logan's joy over this was almost as great as Andrew's.

A series of luncheons and dinners followed with each of the groups, organizations, and men and women in touch with the Logans and Johnsons, basking in the warmth of their combined effort to launch the promising young man from Korea towards Harvard Medical School. Andrew was happiest of all sensing that he was considered by both the Logans and Johnsons as a member of their own individual families.

Before the beginning of classes at Harvard Medical School, Andrew traveled to Chicago to visit a former classmate from

Korea attending college there. After a short visit, he was to re-board a Greyhound Bus to Boston to take up his residence at Vanderbilt Hall at Harvard Medical School. The footlocker had been forwarded ahead allowing him to travel more lightly with a single suitcase, the one he had traveled with from Korea.

CHAPTER 10: HARVARD AND THE GIRL FROM HAWAII

At Vanderbilt Hall, the Medical School dormitory at Harvard, the room he was assigned to was located on the 5th floor. As no elevator was available for use by the occupants of the dormitory, he had to climb the five flights of stairs with his suitcase in tow.

This was easily accomplished whereas the footlocker awaiting him in storage would be another matter. It was too heavy to negotiate up the stairs. Carting its contents by armloads, he was reminded of the generosity of the ladies of the Women's Club of the Episcopal Church in Spartanburg, S.C.

The Hall was bustling with students preparing for the start of classes. Everyone was friendly and he quickly befriended several fellows right away. They came from New York, Oklahoma, Nebraska, Tennessee, and everywhere else it seemed for one student who, while he was born in China of merchant parents, was not Chinese at all, but had lived in many states, the latest in Illinois. Meals at the Hall were exciting, not for the fare but for the interactions with friends that occurred over meals.

Once classes started, a routine was necessary to preset study times and social activities. Andrew worked hard, succeeding in maintaining excellence in every one of his classes.

Not entirely a bookworm though, he also attended various social activities at the Medical School in Boston, at the Cambridge campus of Harvard across the Charles River, and at other colleges around the greater Boston metropolitan area.

One of his former classmates from Kyonggi High School, Harry Cho, had enrolled at the Massachusetts Institute of Technology in Cambridge, and they quickly found each other.

In April, Andrew heard of a gathering of students from Hawaii to be held at Harvard College in Cambridge. He dated a student of Chinese ancestry from one of the colleges in Boston and planned to take her there. He had been told that most of the attendees would likely be of Asian descent, Hawaiians were quite friendly, and he looked forward to a good evening.

They arrived somewhat early at the college and settled down in the lobby awaiting others. A newspaper had been left on the table at the other end of the couch from where they sat. Andrew moved over to read it, reseating himself at the opposite end of the couch, whereas his date remained seated.

As other students entered the area, he noticed their informal dress contrasted sharply with the brown suit and the decidedly mature-looking matching vest he had selected to wear from the largesse of wearables the good ladies of the Episcopal Church in Spartanburg had presented him with.

Oh, well, he thought, we'll only spend a few more minutes and be on our way. No one should notice.

Soon a tall, slender Asian woman with her hair pulled back and pinned in a bun, just like his Mother had worn her hair, entered the room. She smiled and sat on a chair nearby, about midway between the two.

From his dress, she had assumed that he was middle-aged, probably part-Chinese, part-Hawaiian, and that the young lady was either his wife or someone not acquainted with him, because of the apparent absence of active social interaction and the physical distance between them.

After awkward introductions, Andrew learned that the new arrival was of Korean ancestry, born of Korean immigrants in Hawaii. She was an intern at the Children's Hospital Medical Center, Harvard's Pediatric Hospital, right next to the Medical School on Longwood Avenue.

Not long after, the intern excused herself to join the gathering crowd in the main hall where she expected to meet a friend coming from New York, a fellow Hawaiian, she said. So, she bid him goodbye and wished him good luck in his studies and left.

Later that evening, as Andrew was preparing to leave, he put on his outer coat and sought the intern amidst the crowd in the central hall, with his date lagging behind. Finding her, he bid her goodbye, to the surprise of both the intern as well as his date.

During the following week, Andrew sought a meeting with the intern by telephone. His first tries found her too busy or on-call at the hospital. Finally, she agreed to join him for dinner the coming Saturday.

On that Saturday, Andrew donned the blue-gray suit that Mrs. Johnson had had tailored for him, which did not come with a vest. Looking through his small collection of ties, he selected one, tied it before the mirror on his bureau and wondered about Ellen, the intern from Hawaii. He was attracted to her, not because of her Korean-like appearance, or the way she wore her hair, but for undefined reasons. Well, I'll get to know her better he assured himself and set off to meet her.

Just across the street and down a bit was the quarters for the house staff of the Children's Hospital. He rang the bell for the young lady doctor and waited in the small hall at the bottom of the stairway.

Upstairs, Ellen tried to recall what Andrew looked like, but could only remember the brown suit and vest draped over a middle-aged man with a decidedly part-Polynesian appearance.

When she descended and reached the ground floor, she was surprised to find a lean, handsome, tall young man dressed in a dapper suit without a vest—a totally different person than the one she could recall meeting in Cambridge in the much more mature looking brown-vested suit. His hair was dark and wavy, his eyelids were creased over large, piercing, dark eyes flanking a tall aquiline nose perched over somewhat generous, well-shaped lips.

Could this be the same middle-aged man I had spoken to for just a few moments a short time ago, Ellen wondered? Why, he looks completely different! So much for the "costume" he wore, she chuckled to herself.

After greeting each other rather formally, they left by foot towards the tramline launching into light chatter about progress in medical school, the weather, and everything in between. It was only a short ride punctuated with intermittent light conversation before they reached the fifth stop and ascended a flight of stairs to a Japanese restaurant, a rarity in Boston.

He ordered for the two of them. When the order arrived, he proceeded to eat like he was used to, nimbly with chopsticks. To his surprise, she too was nimble with chopsticks.

The rest of the evening was spent in a local pub nearby where the background music was quiet but lively and the guests were clearly largely made up of college-aged students. Andrew drew out a pack of cigarettes, offered one to her, which she declined, and proceeded to puff away, still engaged in conversation. He said he much preferred pipe smoking, but that he had left his pipe behind because it was too bulky and required carting other paraphernalia.

After the evening was spent, they walked back through the

park running the length of the Avenue Louis Pasteur. It had become quite chilly. They draped her coat over both of them and walked closely together with their arms locked. At the end of the Avenue, they entered the lobby of Vanderbilt Hall, his dormitory, to chat and warm themselves.

Now they got into family histories and Andrew asked her if she knew of his Grandfather, Choi Nam Sun or Yukdang. To his disappointment, she said she did not. At this point, he wondered about her knowledge of anything of significance in Korean history. However, as he proceeded to inform her of some of his Grandfather's accomplishments, she recognized him as the patriot about whom she was well acquainted by deed, not by name.

He had drafted what later became the Declaration of Independence for Korea at the time of the non-violent uprising against the Japanese. The uprising was cruelly squelched and many of the insurgents were killed, but not Choi Nam Sun. She was delighted that Andrew was his grandson and the conversation continued into the late evening.

Before long it was time to leave for the intern's quarters. At parting, each experienced a peculiar sense of loneliness. Both wished the evening could last forever. Andrew knew he was not the same as before this meeting. Finally after promising to continue to see each other, they parted.

A series of weekend meetings followed, tying the bond between them even tighter. Finals came and went for him without difficulty. Rotations from one clinic to another kept the intern busy. Each looked forward eagerly to their next meeting.

However, not everything was rosy between the two, as might be expected. She was a Roman Catholic, and while he insisted this made no difference, he often argued over some of Catholicism's fundamental edicts and precepts. The Virgin Mary was revered to an idolatrous level and the absolution of sins by the mere recitation of prayers following a confessional admission to a priest seemed to him to be impediments to a primary relationship with God. They discussed and argued points for many hours without apparent success in swaying either to the other's point of view.

One summer evening, Andrew formally proposed marriage producing a ring set with a small diamond from his pocket. The price of the ring had eaten substantially into his assets, but he had been prudent, purchasing a modest one with the largest stone for the price he was prepared to shell out.

She accepted his proposal on the condition the marriage be a Catholic one, not to be broken except by death, and he agreed to these terms while vowing to continue to worship as an Anglican.

Discussions about other matters naturally arose from time to time during the engagement period. For example, the eventual choice of residence for them was an issue discussed at great length and with deep feelings without resolution. He insisted that they would live in Korea following completion of his medical training, pointing out that this had always been his primary intent, that he needed to meet his family obligations as head of the Kangs to be physically present amongst the members of the clan, and that he had a desire to contribute to the needs of his own country.

She raised the issue of her identity with America, her ignorance of many things Korean, her rejection of the manner by which women were kept subservient to men in Korea, her inability to see how she could practice medicine in a primarily male dominated society, and so forth.

Thus, she resisted his adamant insistence that they eventually take up permanent residence in Korea. After much expenditure of emotional energy on this matter, each expecting God to lead the other to his/her preference for a place of residence, they finally agreed to circumvent the stumbling issue, proceeding instead with plans for their marriage, the initial step necessary to forge their lives together.

Andrew wrote a letter to Ellen's parents outlining his lineage and requesting their permission to marry their daughter.

He also contacted Uncle Choi Han Woong informing him of his choice of a bride and asking for his blessing of the marriage.

One long weekend, he took a bus back to Spartanburg to discuss his decision to marry with Mr. Logan.

For Andrew, everyone agreed to his choice and sent their blessings. By contrast, everyone in Ellen's family strongly disapproved of the marriage, threatening to cut off all further contact with her should she go through with it. This was an unsettling matter for the two, who were unaware of the basis for their objection.

Later, they learned that Ellen's relatives considered Andrew to be one of a number of opportunistic Korean men who sought to marry vulnerable Korean-American women in order to fulfill immigration requirements to win entry into the U.S. Apparently, a number of naive Korean-American women in Hawaii had become just such victims and her folks were convinced the young man from Korea was making marital overtures to their daughter for the same reason. The possibility that the two young people had truly fallen in love and wanted to commit themselves to each other for the rest of their lives had not entered into their minds. Ellen had informed them of the lack of regard Andrew had for gaining citizenship and his insistence on returning to Korea to live after his training, which posed a dilemma for her. Nothing altered their thinking, however, and before long all further contact was severed by her parents, who ignored her continued correspondence and refused to accept her telephone calls.

Despite this turmoil, wedding plans proceeded for September 6, 1958 to be followed by a small reception for about 40 of their closest friends.

Just prior to the end of Andrew's first year at Harvard Medical School, the Clinical Tutor to whom Andrew had been assigned, Dr. John Decker at the Massachusetts General Hospital (MGH), a gentle giant of a man who was born in China to missionary parents, had informed him of the availability of summer research projects for students completing the freshman year. Dr. Decker referred Andrew to Dr. Tom Hall at the Lemmuel Shattuck Hospital, a Harvard affiliated State Hospital, for possible assignment on a summer project under his direction. This was subsequently arranged. As a trainee in research for the summer in Dr. Hall's laboratory, he would be permitted to continue his residence at Vanderbilt Hall.

To bolster the small salary he would be receiving, he signed on for an evening job as a Clinical Laboratory technician for the summer, to be on-call at the Boston-Lying-In Hospital located just across the rotary in front of Vanderbilt Hall.

As the summer wore on, Andrew and Ellen continued to work out the details of the wedding squeezing in visits to potential living sites for their life together, to second-hand furniture stores for the best buys with their meager funds, to the printer for invitations, to caterers for the best price for a small reception, to a florist, to rental units for appropriate attire for Andrew and the best man, and to wedding shops to purchase appropriate gowns for Ellen and her attendant.

While they only had a small budget to work with, the delight they both took in the selection of items and terms for purchase or rental gave them the illusion that the plans might have been for a prince and his princess in disguise, not the two hard-working, underpaid (none in Ellen's case) and overworked medical trainees that they were.

CHAPTER 11: RUDE ENCOUNTER WITH ARTHRITIS

Approximately two weeks before the wedding, Andrew felt the insidious development of pain in the neck and back, which grew in intensity over a few days and was accompanied by a sense of generalized malaise and the appearance of a moderate fever. Later, joint pains developed in the wrists and ankles without known trauma to these particular joints. Within a couple of days, he could barely sit upright, let alone turn his head from side to side. Years earlier, while yet in Korea, he had several bouts of somewhat painful discomfort affecting the same areas. The discomfort he had then would subside after a few days without increasing in intensity, unlike what developed this time around, which persisted.

Ellen accompanied him during a hastily arranged visit with the Harvard Medical Student Health Physician at the Peter Bent Brigham Hospital. The diagnostic workup including x-rays of the spine led to the diagnosis of acute spondylo-arthritis, or arthritis of the spine. The physician recommended immediate hospitalization for rest and the use of aspirin as treatment for this condition as commonly prescribed in America.

Hospitalization was refused by Andrew. He insisted that if oral medication and bed rest were the means to quiet the arthritis, he could accomplish both without hospitalization.

Ellen did her best to have him reconsider the matter, fully cognizant that there was no means to physically care for him in his incapacitated state outside of the hospital. She assured him that letters of postponement of the wedding could be sent without difficulty.

"No, I will not be hospitalized! Treat me as an outpatient, instead," he demanded.

Frustrated, the internist said that he recommended hospitalization in order to give his joints a rest, something unlikely to be achieved outside of the hospital, especially as Andrew lived in the dormitory requiring physical exercise to cope with the basic necessities of life. However, if he insisted, he could remain not hospitalized with aspirin as the drug of choice in his outpatient management for rheumatoid arthritis, the doctor finally conceded.

Perplexed, Ellen seriously questioned Andrew's judgment regarding hospitalization, but found no reward in arguing with him about the matter. He would not be hospitalized, period!

Elasticized bandages were used to restrain motion of the painful joints of the wrist and ankles and he returned to his room at Vanderbilt Hall, negotiating the five flights of steps slowly and with great care, with Ellen beside him.

Andrew's laboratory chief, Dr. Tom Hall, a kindly personable man, came by to see him the next day, alarmed by the complaint of back pain and physical disability given as the reason for his absence from work during their telephone conversation. Dr. Hall feared the possibility of meningitis.

The good doctor dropped by the dormitory to examine Andrew and was relieved that no signs of meningitis were present. Seeing the pain the young medical student was suffering, he recommended that Dr. Ellis Dresner come by to see him at the dormitory and arranged such a visit.

Dr. Dresner was the researcher in the adjoining laboratory and Andrew had come to know him in person. He was a rheumatologist from England and was conducting research to understand the basis for acute non-infectious arthritis.

Soon after, Dr. Dresner did come to Vanderbilt Hall just to see Andrew. He carefully examined Andrew and agreed with the diagnosis of ankylosing spondylo-arthritis. He explained the therapeutic strategy he would use. Having been trained in England and had considerable experience with phenylbuta-zone, a drug not used to any significant extent in the U.S., but the preferred drug of choice by rheumatologists in England, he said he would recommend treatment with that very drug, phenylbutazone.

Treatment with phenylbutazone could result in a devastating depression of the bone marrow, wiping out red and white blood cells as well as platelet formation with dangerous consequences, he cautioned, which was the reason for its not being used in the U.S. But, it was a powerful drug, reversing the effects of arthritis in the majority of patients without the marrow effects. He recommended this drug, certain that careful monitoring of the peripheral blood cells could lead to the timely detection of the slightest evidence of bone marrow depression at which point the drug could be withdrawn without permanent damage. And, Andrew concurred with the treatment proposed by Dr. Dresner.

To monitor the marrow, blood tests would have to be done on a regular basis necessitating a trip to the laboratory. This posed a considerable challenge. Excruciating joint pains constrained movement from his room at Vanderbilt Hall to almost everywhere else, let alone up and down the five flights of stairs. A change was necessary and a temporary second floor site was located for him in the communal living room of the house staff quarters where Ellen was living at the hospital nearby with agreement from each of the other residents of the quarters, all of whom had come to know Andrew quite well.

Almost within days after the start of phenylbutazone, the pain began to lessen enabling him to hobble short distances using crutches fitted under his armpits. However, he could only sit upright for a short time, having to lie flat on his back within 10-15 minutes of sitting.

Despite his almost immediate initial response to phenylbutazone, improvement did not continue as rapidly thereafter. However, plans for the wedding were left unchanged at Andrew's adamant insistence. Several days before the wedding date, Andrew moved from the house staff quarters into the apartment on Longwood Avenue, which they had leased to be their first home together after their marriage.

Classmates from medical school and his old friend from Korea, Peter Lee, who came all the way to Boston from Pittsburgh where he was a student at the University of Pittsburgh, helped with the move, staying with him, and taking care of his necessities. Peter was to be the Best Man at the wedding.

On the wedding day, Ellen dressed in her cramped quarters together with her fellow intern, Gertrude (Trudi) Muersett, from Zurich, Switzerland, her Maid of Honor. At the right hour, the two were driven to the Catholic Church by the pediatrician, Dr. William Dorsey, and his wife from Beverly, Massachusetts. Dr. Dorsey had been her Attending Physician during her rotation through Beverly Hospital and he had agreed to walk the bride down the aisle.

Andrew's friends, Carl Engleman, who was an upper classman of Andrew's at Harvard, Gordie Robb, a classmate, and the Best Man, Peter Lee, dressed him in a rented tuxedo, maneuvered him down the stairs of the apartment house, and drove him to the Church. There they led him through the back door and propped him up front on crutches to await his bride-to-be. Dressed in the rented tuxedo complete with a black silk cummerbund, he was a handsome groom, indeed, watching the slow approach of his bride-to-be towards the altar on the arm of Dr. Dorsey.

There, Andrew vowed to love and honor Ellen and she did likewise vow to love and honor Andrew, 'til death did them part.

After the ceremony, Tiger walked haltingly down the hall leaning on his crutches with his bride at his side. He was hurting with every step. He stood at the door of the beautiful Cathedral to greet his friends, supported by the pair of crutches, and even stood for a few portraits to be taken. Later, he was driven to the reception where a wheel chair awaited him.

As the celebration reached the mid-point, a toast for happiness, long life, and good health was offered by the Best Man, Peter Lee.

By the time the wedding reception was over, Andrew was pale and sweaty from the pain he suffered enduring the whole event in an upright position, placing undue and continuous pressure on his inflamed joints. Finally, returning to the apartment with help from the same friends, he lay flat on his back in great relief!

The Best Man, the Maid of Honor, and one of Andrew's former Wofford classmates joined in the small wedding dinner, which was held in the apartment serving take-out Chinese from a corner Mom & Pop diner.

And so, Andrew and Ellen were married, marking the start of a new chapter in his life. Now, Tiger had a companion with whom to share new experiences and challenges.

Over time they learned much about each other, but it would take many, many years before he could unlock the area of his brain harboring the images of that dreaded experience of searching for and finding his beloved Mother as a mutilated corpse with her facial expression revealing the terror and horror she was undergoing at the moment of death.

Within days of the wedding, sophomore medical school classes began with Andrew unable to physically attend. For a month, he tried to keep up with the lessons at home, reading all assignments and lecture notes, which his good buddies, Bill Ellis, Jim Warram, Gene Di-Cero, and Lubert Stryer, collected and brought by to him on a regular basis. In a valiant effort to keep up with the work, Andrew would read lying flat on his back with his eyes trained on the text wedged between the bars under the large hospital feeding tray raised to its maximum. From time to time, he would roll over onto his tummy with the upper half of his face extended over the bed so that his eyes could peer down at the open textbook on the floor. A small lamp was used to light the passages he poured over, tilted up or down, depending on whether he was on his back or on his tummy.

Day after day he studied, hoping to keep up while he healed sufficiently to return to class. Finally, after more than a month had passed, Andrew came to the realization that he would not be able to return for the-02 year because of the unremitting nature of his arthritis.

Just before the Christmas break, Andrew's former classmates, Bill Ellis, Jim Warram, and Dick Lamb, knocked on the door in surprise to both Andrew and Ellen with a Christmas tree, complete with lights and decorations, a wreath, wine, a holiday record, and lots of good cheer. Ellen wheeled Andrew to join in the festivity of setting up the Christmas decorations. Each of his buddies would from time to time ask Andrew whether this or that bulb looked better here or there, engaging him actively in these efforts, making him an active participant. In the meantime, Ellen quickly prepared a meal for all on the fly, so to speak.

When the tiny apartment was fully decorated, they all sat down to eat and enjoy the holiday cheer. For the first time since his illness, Andrew managed to sit up in the wheel chair for a couple of hours instead of the usual fifteen minutes per meal. He was obviously reveling in the warmth and spontaneity of his fellowship with his friends as well as the joy of the season.

This occasion heralded the beginning of his healing, whether prompted or not by the goodwill and cheer his friends had brought, cannot be said, of course. Over the next few weeks, gradual improvement was clearly noticeable. Fortunately, no signs of marrow depression had been detected throughout his treatment with phenylbutazone.

Progressively recovering sufficiently to move around nimbly on crutches, he sought and obtained an interim job working in research under Dr. Ellis Dresner in February of 1959 at the Lemuel Shattuck Hospital in Jamaica Plain, at the outskirts of Boston.

He spent the rest of the academic year there, acquiring the background and basic laboratory skills that fed a growing interest in the pathological and biochemical understanding of the basis of rheumatoid arthritis, or R.A., of which ankylosing-spondylitis was then thought to be a form localized in the spinous tissues. The fact that the basis for this disease was not known intrigued him and he soon recognized the great variety of routes that could be taken to investigate R.A.

The clinical project undertaken with Dr. Dresner was to determine the presence or not of collagenase activity in the synovial fluid of patients with R.A. In the face of histopathological findings of degradation of collagenous matter in the joints of patients with R.A., it was logical to consider a role for the enzyme involved in the degradation of collagen, collagenase. Ordinarily, collagenase activity was not found in normal synovial fluid, ergo no matter the circumstance(s) leading to its possible appearance in the fluid bathing the joints, the presence of collagenase in synovial fluid would support a role for collagenase in the damage done to the joint collagen, Dresner reasoned.

In order to set up the test for the enzyme, collagen had to be extracted and purified before it could be used as the substrate in an assay for collagenase, since purified collagen was not yet available on the scientific market.

The scientific paper Andrew was to follow was published by Dr. Jerome Gross of the Massachusetts General Hospital, or the MGH. Purified tropocollagen, the soluble form of collagen, added to various aliquots of synovial fluid collected from patients would demonstrate a reduction in viscosity upon degradation of the tropocollagen by collagenase, if the enzyme were present in the synovial fluid. Nearly a dozen patient samples had been obtained for testing, but no significant change in viscosity was found. Eventually, an abstract was published on their negative finding.

A number of years later, Dr. Ted Harris published on work done at the National Institutes of Health (NIH) where synovial fluids from a far larger group of patients showed that only about 10 percent of samples from R.A. patients reduced the viscosity of tropocollagen to indicate the presence of collagenase activity in those particular samples.

Thus, in retrospect, if the number of patients had been expanded many fold in Dr. Dresner's and Andrew's study, a more positive finding might have resulted to indicate the presence of collagenase activity in about 10 percent of affected patients. As it was later discovered, collagenase itself appears to be present in joint fluid, but its activity is unexpressed owing to the presence of a tissue inhibitor of metalloproteinase activity or TIMP, and the regulation of the interactions of TIMP and collagenase activity is disturbed in about 10 percent of affected patients who exhibit collagenase activity.

This was Andrew's initial effort in research on rheumatoid arthritis. While their finding was a negative one, his interest had been aroused and would not be diverted from learning the hidden facts about the biology and pathogenesis of rheumatoid arthritis—the disease, which hurt him and stymied his educational plans.

CHAPTER 12: FAMILY AND CAREER SHAPING

After the passage of a year since he was rudely afflicted with the severe bout of arthritis and a couple of weeks before he was slated to finally return to medical school, their first child was born on August 18, 1959.

She was tiny, beautiful, and hungry as evident by her eagerness at the breast. Why, she only weighed slightly over six pounds and needed to catch up to the average for babies, which was seven pounds, Ellen would say, unawares that the baby's weight was average for Asians, as reported later in the pediatric literature.

Prior to her arrival, they had agreed that Ellen would select her English first name and Andrew would select a Korean middle name for the baby. She was called Cynthia Hyun Ok (Wise Ruby) Kang. According to Andrew, Hyun or Wise would serve as the base name for other children God would give them, as was customary in Korea.

At first, both parents centered their activities around the baby's schedule, tip-toeing around to keep the squeaky floors of the old apartment house from waking their baby, who was endowed with especially keen auditory sensors.

Before long, Andrew learned to study with the baby playing in his lap or fussing over his ears, his hair and even the papers or opened book on the desk where he sat trying to read and digest the lessons of his biomedical courses. He was baby-sitting after supper, while his wife saw to the daily diaper rinsing/washing and formula preparations for the next day after a full day at the hospital for her. She was still in clinical training as a resident at the Children's Hospital and the baby spent her days in the care of another medical student's wife for the first several months before a nanny was engaged.

When Ellen was ready to relieve Andrew, she frequently found the baby asleep in his arms, as he continued in his concentrated study over books or papers propped up before him.

He rarely relinquished the baby without a juicy kiss on her cheek, often causing the baby to wake in a startle. Startled though she was, the baby would find her dear Daddy peering at her, whereupon she would fall back to sleep, reassured that he was nearby.

Financially, they were below the poverty line with the two of them living solely off of Andrew's meager earnings in the laboratory where he continued to work on the weekends. Postgraduate medical trainees were not paid a wage at the Children's Hospital Medical Center and at many other centers in the 60's. Crucially about this time, Ellen's family had reopened communication with the couple, and one of her brothers, Henry, had agreed to help them through their difficult times with a monthly payment to cover the rental with some to spare. With this support, they could see the completion of Ellen's training, assured that a salaried position would follow.

Andrew worked in the laboratory of Dr. Melvin Glimcher in the Orthopedic Department at the MGH during the summer after completion of his sophomore year. The work concerned the study of ossification of bone, specifically to determine whether activation of ATPase was an initial step in the nucleation of calcium phosphate. After a quarter of hard work, the thesis was not supported by their findings and no publication resulted.

The third and fourth years of medical school came and went rapidly. Andrew concentrated on his studies and home life, relinquishing part-time work.

All the while, his daughter grew and matured, reaching her mile stones much earlier than generally expected, to the joy of her parents. Interestingly, she never crawled, preferring to stand and walk instead shortly after learning to sit up for extended periods without back support.

About that time, his wife completed her training and began a research fellowship in the Department of Neurology, bringing in some badly needed income.

In 1962, he graduated from Harvard Medical School. Earlier, he had been elected to Alpha Omega Alpha, the honorary society for medical students. At the graduation ceremony, his wife was caught completely by surprise when his name was called to receive the M.D. degree Magna Cum Laude. She had often worried that his level of concentration might not have been optimal because he had to share in the care of the baby to the extent that he had. She was unable to stem the flow of joyful tears streaking down both cheeks on seeing him rise to receive this honor. As she dabbed her eyes and cheeks and blew her nose, little Cynthia looked up at her Mother and asked, "What happened, Mommy? Why are you crying?"

She answered, "It's your Daddy, Cynthia. He is such a wonder to me!"

He was accepted for training in Internal Medicine at the Peter Bent Brigham Hospital in Boston.

The family had already moved to Francis Street to a third floor flat located across the parking lot of the Brigham Hospital.

Sometime before he began his internship, he launched on the building of the first of a long list of home-carpentered products to come. He had never carpentered before. With the most elemental of tools, he fashioned a sandbox for Cynthia, sandpapering it with care to remove all splinters and painting it a warm rose. Promptly filled with clean sand, it saw extensive use perched on the back porch next to the high railing of their rented apartment.

In September of the first of his clinical training years at the Peter Bent Brigham Hospital in Boston, they had a second child, another daughter, just about the same in weight as Cynthia was, a bit over six pounds. She was born with a head full of black, wavy hair, whereas Cynthia's pate at birth had been covered with only a light growth of soft fuzz. The newborn shared the same enthusiasm at the breast as her sister Cynthia had at birth. She was named Edith Hyun Ju (Wise Pearl) Kang.

Edith soon learned to crawl long distances, peering from one room to another in search of Cynthia, to share whatever she had been given gripped tightly in her fist, while maneuvering forward on all four extremities. On finding Cynthia, she would offer the treasure she held in her fist, be it a bun (now squished), a cookie (now crumbled), a banana (now squashed), or a toy (the only thing intact), to Cynthia's horror. A squeamish call for help was all that was needed to bring the Nanny or her parents to Cynthia's "defense," which was invariably followed by an immediate exercise of washing both Cynthia's and Edith's hands as well as mopping the trail that the baby had blazed marking her scouting route.

Now, pressure was brought on Andrew to consider getting a permanent resident's visa (Green Card). "Our children are American citizens; so am I. There should be no doubt about our need to be in a safe part of the world. Furthermore, you must continue to be with us under all circumstances, not far off in Korea," Ellen would nag, reopening the issue of their permanent country of residence.

Eventually, he agreed and filed the necessary papers to obtain a Permanent Resident's Visa.

The war in Vietnam had developed in the interim and according to law, all Green Card holders would be subject to the Draft. Soon, doctors were being called up for Selective Service. According to the Recruiting Office Sergeant, Andrew would not qualify as an officer because he was not a U.S. citizen. If drafted, he would be a foot soldier, no matter his medical education and training.

Consequently, he proceeded with filing for citizenship, which was granted soon thereafter.

About this time, the National Institutes of Health (NIH) announced a Research Associate Program where a designee would be an officer of the United States Public Health Service (USPHS), fulfilling U.S. Selective Service obligations. A listing of the laboratories open for such Research Associates was scanned to select a suitable NIH laboratory for possible continuation of research in R.A.

Andrew applied for a position with Dr. Karl Piez at the Dental Institute. Dr. Piez was deciphering the structure of collagen—a fundamental approach and a logical place to continue preparation for future work, Tiger, or Andrew, thought. Fortunately, he was inducted as a Lt. Commander in the USPHS at the NIH to work in Dr. Karl Piez's laboratory in Bethesda, Maryland in lieu of service in the U.S. Army.

At that time, Andrew had not fully completed his training in Internal Medicine, requiring one additional year to qualify for Boards in Internal Medicine. Under the pressure of the Vietnam War, postgraduate medical training places were going unfilled as physicians were being inducted to serve in the armed forces. His appointment as a Lt. Commander in the USPHS at the NIH was regarded as a service obligation and arrangements to hold the last year of clinical training open for him to complete after his tour of duty was over was readily made.

Ellen had acquired a position with the Department of Health, Education and Welfare as a Consultant in Metabolic Diseases.

Together, Andrew, his wife and their two children searched areas in the Washington, D.C. perimeter for a home to rent or lease, based on the educational programs offered by the various communities surrounding the capital city of America. Montgomery County in Maryland was their choice and Bethesda was ideal from the standpoint of its location for both of them and for its outstanding record in public education.

They leased a country house set on a large estate bordering the home of the owner. Across the street were comfortable homes for many NIH workers and the house was only two blocks away from Grosvenor Elementary School, easily accessible to his first-born daughter for kindergarten and first grade the following year.

Moving from an apartment in Boston without a yard to care for to a lease hold with a rather large one was a decided challenge to Andrew. But, one of the first things he set out to do was to build another sandbox, larger than the first one, where his children were to spend many, many happy hours together and with their friends from the neighborhood. Innovatively, he added a work-shelf to this one giving his children a worktable for more stable mountains, animal shapes, and cakes to fashion during their play. He added another feature to protect his children from the droppings of birds and the neighborhood cats—a wooden lid that covered the entire sandbox which matched the box itself in color, a beautiful deep red.

Mowing the yard was a mega chore, especially with the antiquated, industrial-sized machine that came with the lease. Each turn cut a huge swath, requiring Andrew to use all of his strength to keep the machine from swerving in a circle. He did the yard work on his own taking the precaution of clearing the yard of the poison ivy which abounded, especially in areas his daughters tended to brush against in their hilariously joyous antics on the back lawn with their good friends from across the way.

One experience that he was glad was unlikely to repeat itself was with a snake all curled up around the fuse box. It was dusk and the lights had gone out, not because of the bulb but more likely because of a burnt fuse. In the basement, the snake was equally as startled as Andrew was, but was prepared to challenge him than give up it's apparent comfort nestled over and around the suspended fuse box.

Needless to say, Andrew won and the lights returned forthwith!

Andrew was extremely productive in Dr. Karl Piez's laboratory, not only with the amount of work he accomplished but from what he learned and the contacts he was able to make. The many collaborative interactions Dr. Piez had with others around the country as well as others at the NIH impressed him. It enlarged his view of what one could accomplish in research.

Together with Piez, Gross, Nagai, Martin, Bornstein, and Miller, he had numerous publications in the scientific literature after his two years of service. The work centered on the structure of collagen, the nature and localization of intra-molecular cross-linkages, the use of specific enzymes to effect limited and reproducible segments of collagen, and the amino acid sequences of the resulting peptides.

Dr. Jerome (Jerry) Gross from the MGH in Boston came down to Dr. Piez's laboratory for consultation and interaction on a number of occasions. Eventually, arrangements were made for Andrew to join Dr. Gross' laboratory at the MGH for a Postdoctoral Fellowship upon completion of the third year of his Internal Medicine residency at the Peter Bent Brigham Hospital in Boston following completion of his work with Dr. Piez.

Two months prior to the end of Andrew's tour of duty, a third child arrived, another daughter. As with her sisters, she too weighed just slightly over six pounds. Like her older sister Cynthia, she only wore a light fuzz on her head, not the mop of curly hair that Edith was born with. Peering at her Mother with her large eyes opened, almost from the moment of her birth, she seemed to be asking what the ruckus was all about. Later, she would often stop in the middle of suckling and peer into the feeder's face as if to ask, "Who are you?"

They named her Audrey Hyun Duk (Wise and Virtuous) Kang.

Each of her sisters took some interest in the baby who watched and gurgled with wonder at the countless movements per unit time that surrounded the appearance of Cynthia's and/or Edith's form(s) within her field of vision.

Taking advantage of the proximity of major landmark Governmental sites of importance, not only historically but also from their beauty and elegance, Tiger took his family to visit the major sites in Washington, D.C. The Smithsonian Museum, the Space Museum, and Washington's wonderful Zoo were visited innumerable times, with each visit as engaging to the children as to their parents.

The two years in Bethesda where both were salaried gave them the financial boost they needed for an upgrade in life. Andrew kept the financial accounting, managing to save enough for a down payment on a modest home in an educationally superb community in one of the townships of Newton, Massachusetts called Waban.

And so, they returned to Massachusetts having selected a neighborhood filled with other young families with children eager to learn, play, and exchange friendship. The elementary school was nearby, as were the library and the church, Episcopal, of course.

As he had promised after an extended discussion regarding the religious upbringing and education of their children, which he had evidently won, Andrew saw to the proper timing of their baptism, confirmation and education in the Episcopalian manner.

No matter where they lived, he quickly located a place of worship, which suited everyone. One or two visits and a place would be identified where the family registered and attended as communicants.

Following completion of his last year of Internal Medicine training at the Peter Bent Brigham Hospital, Andrew joined Dr. Jerry Gross at the MGH as a Postdoctoral Fellow. At the same time, his clinical experience was with Dr. Steven Krane through the Rheumatology Clinic at the MGH.

His first application for extramural research support was made to the Arthritis Foundation and the NIH. Both were to be awarded and he had to choose between the two granting agencies. The Arthritis Foundation award was for five years whereas the NIH's was for three years, so naturally, he opted for the Arthritis Foundation.

Andrew worked hard and collaborated with others in Dr. Gross' laboratory and with investigators in other laboratories in the Boston area and the NIH. Over the span of the five years, he accomplished highly significant and spectacular work, all documented by an impressive number of publications appearing in first rank journals. He was clearly a rising researcher in the field of connective tissue biology and pathobiology.

Among the works he had accomplished included the identification of the site of action of tadpole collagenase, precisely defining the site at residue 775-776, at glycine-leucine or glycine isoleucine, making a single cleavage through all three chains of the triple helix retaining the triple helical structure.

Tadpole collagenase was later to be referred to as matrix metalloproteinase 1, or MMP 1. Cleavage through all three chains of the helix turns out to be the general model followed by other collagenases on other types of collagen, although at different specific bonds. And, it is the triple helical configuration of collagen that renders collagen resistant to the action of general proteases.

This was the first time the physiological mechanism of collagen degradation was elucidated and subsequently the pathological role of this and other related enzymes could open the way for new areas of study.

This seminal work enabled the completion of the amino acid sequences of Type I collagen and also of substantial portions of Type II and Type III collagen by both Dr. Kang and other contributors. These findings formed the basis for the structure-function studies that he and his coworkers were subsequently to pursue.

Other accomplishments from this period included defining the relationships between inter and intramolecular cross-links and the effect of renaturation and in vitro formation of cross-links; description of the high degree of heterogeneity amongst the several types of collagen along with the presence of carbohydrate moieties in linkage with various amino acid residues; early studies on the specificity of bacterial collagenase; and demonstration of the ability of embryonic spinal cord epithelium to synthesize collagen in vitro.

Nearing the end of the research-funding period, he wrote another NIH application and asked for the maximum salary they would allow, $25,000 per year. With his family of three growing children, he had received approval from Dr. Gross to list that amount in his application.

About the time the application was to be processed for mailing to the NIH, he was informed that the Department of Medicine Chairman would not sign off because the salary requested exceeded the $22,000 limit set for comparable positions at the MGH.

This was upsetting to Andrew who had just run into his classmate and fellow trainee at the MGH, Dr. Ted Harris, who was leaving for Dartmouth, New Hampshire.

"Look around, Andy, there's plenty of other places to find work that pays," Harris advised.

Furthermore, a former fellow resident at the Brigham who had maintained contact with him, Dr. Larry Kedes, had recently moved from Boston to Stanford University as an independent researcher. His more recent commentary to Andrew raised the issue of what he was doing at the MGH where he had no private space and no independent status.

And so, Andrew discretely contacted Dr. John Decker, his former Medical School mentor who had moved to the NIH, inquiring of his knowledge of positions elsewhere, informing him of the salary constraints being imposed at the MGH, the growing needs of his family, as well as his wish to be able to expand and grow as an independent researcher.

Not long after, six invitations came to Andrew for consideration. Emotionally in a turmoil considering his attachment to Boston and the happiness of his family in their present environment, he nevertheless followed up on each of them.

Among the several institutions he visited, he selected the University of Tennessee in Memphis (UT) because the position would allow him independence and room for growth and was linked to a Veterans' Hospital for additional laboratory support and growth. And, the move would satisfy the financial needs of his family, both at that time and in the coming years to come, especially with regard to his children's eventual college education.

Dr. Gross and others tried in vain to convince him that he was making a serious error in judgment, certain the move would stymie the progression of his already promising career. Several even suggested he had temporarily lost his mind for giving up an Associate Professorship at Harvard Medical School for a Professorship anywhere else, they said trying in vain to get him to change his mind.

He was cocksure though, with no doubt that he would continue to be productive and successful, no matter where he went. After all, success or not was dependent as much on the hard work he knew he could put out, not merely a reflection of the reputation of one's surroundings. Thus, he forged ahead with the move.

CHAPTER 13: BACK TO THE SOUTH

The family left Boston in the summer of 1972 in a new Ford Country Squire station wagon, driving over the Blue Ridge Mountains, headed southwestward to a city along the Mississippi River, smack in the middle of the continent. With their children and last minute household goods and their pet canary, Pecky, cram-packed, they arrived to settle at Massey Road in Memphis, Tennessee. However, not until they had broken the long trip with a memorable visit along the way to the Luray Caverns of southern Virginia.

There in the generous belly of the Cavern stood the stalactite and stalagmite columns produced over millions of years, Andrew told his children, reinforcing in them what he had been instilling regarding the eventual effectiveness of a steady consistent effort toward the formation or attainment of significant results.

Joining Andrew in his move to the University of Tennessee was Dr. Richard Katzman from the MGH. In fact, the moving van was filled with both his and Dick's family household goods when it arrived in Memphis.

Dick had been working on a primitive collagen, separating the ?-chains of the sea anemone at the MGH at the same time as he had been with Dr. Gross. They had consulted with each other on numerous occasions during their individual work.

In Memphis, Andrew had been recruited to head the Rheumatology Section and to serve as the Associate Chief of Staff for Research and Development at the Veterans Administration Hospital (VAH) in Memphis. He was to be a Professor of Medicine at the University of Tennessee (UT) under Dr. Gene Stollerman and was also appointed as an Associate Professor of Biochemistry.

Within a year, he had recruited Dr. Arnold Postlethwaite fresh from a Rheumatology Fellowship at Duke University under Dr. William Kelly. Arnie was to remain as a loyal and steadfast researcher for the duration of Andrew's stay at UT.

Dr. Jerome Seyer joined Andrew two years later. He had been working with Dr. Mel Glimcher at the MGH in Boston where they had previously met under the most unusual circumstances. It seemed that columns required to purify bulk amounts of collagen peptides were never large enough, nor long enough for Dr. Gross' group. Accordingly, Dr. Gross had engaged the cooperation of Dr. Glimcher and the building engineers at the MGH to allow a column with a length long enough to encompass an upright man to span their benchtop all the way up to the ceiling, emerging at the floor of another laboratory's coldroom, one flight above.

Jerry Seyer had the singularly unique experience of stepping onto the trap door of the coldroom floor, which was intended as the top of the long column from below. Fortunately, it was neither filled with resin nor fluid at the time of Jerry's dramatic entry into Andrew's line of vision. He landed onto the benchtop one floor below rather suddenly, making for their immediate acquaintance and launching quite a bit of hilarity among all the laboratory workers located on both floors.

Uninjured though he was, it took two more years before Jerry Seyer considered joining Andrew in Memphis, not only to reconnect with his Missouri roots, one of seven states bordering Tennessee, but also to gain headway in his own effort to decipher the structure of collagen.

In contrast to some dire predictions issued at the time of his decision to leave Boston, Andrew succeeded far more than even he had imagined he would. He recruited other researchers, trained fellows from his own institution as well as from all over the world, all the while expanding his knowledge base and enlarging his laboratory capabilities. He provided a nurturing environment for his recruitees and their collaborators, expending his influence with wisdom and great discretion. All of this was conducive to his success in research, and he made much progress in this regard.

The work on collagenase was extended by the group he assembled in Memphis (Mainardi, Hibbs, Hasty, Crawford, Postlethwaite, Seyer, Stricklin, Hoidal, Reife, Stuart). The isolation and characterization of other MMPs, namely, gelatinase and another human neutrophil collagenase, MMP8, followed. The specific cleavage of human type III collagen by human neutrophil elastase was defined. Interestingly,.by contrast to human type III collagen, the enzyme did not cleave the helical region of human type I or type II collagen.

Clinical studies of the secretory enzymes released by human pulmonary alveolar macrophages during inflammation were performed. Among their secretory repertoire of enzymes are neutral proteinases, including metalloproteinases such as interstitial collagenase, elastase and gelatinase.

Also, after stimulation with macrophage supernatants, human rheumatoid synovial cells themselves, in culture, secrete several distinct metalloproteinases including MMPI, which acts on 5 of 13 known types of collagen and degrades native fibrillar collagen, including gelatinase and stromelysin.

Dr. Kang and his collaborators demonstrated that the three collagen chains run as a heterotrimer the entire length of the molecule. By brute force, they established the complete amino acid sequence of the Al(type I) and the A2(type I) chains which together make up type I collagen. Also, the amino acid sequences of type III collagen, the vast majority of type II collagen, and some portions of type V collagen were similarly determined by the Edman degradation technique, all over the span of some ten years. Importantly, findings made by this laboriously difficult method have been supported by more recent work using DNA techniques.

In parallel to work on the structure of collagen, functional emphasis was given to the role of collagen in the vessels, as a biologically active substrate interacting with connective tissue cells, platelets and the macrophages.

Together with Dick Katzman and Dr. Ed Beachey, the interaction between collagen and human platelets was localized to an active glycopeptide fragment of the alpha chain, Al-CB5.

While his contributions were being recognized world-wide, he continued to nurture his personal family in a multitude of ways. For example, in 1976, he was invited to an International Meeting of Connective Tissue Biology in Munich. He decided to take his entire family with him to visit Europe. Considering their prior debts, their current financial arrangements to cover the looming educational costs for their daughters, and the unimpressive salaries received by academics, he had to borrow to underwrite the costs anticipated. However, he reasoned that in addition to the educational aspects of the trip, a lasting image of the warmth and joy of the family exploring the historical sites abroad together would be imprinted on everyone. Elaborate plans were made for stopovers in Frankfurt, Munich, Zurich,

Venice, Rome, Paris, and side trips to the Alps and Florence by rail and the Island of Capri by boat.

And as he had imagined, memories from that first trip to Europe are still vividly recalled by all members of the family as representing the best trip the family had ever taken together — and there were many, many other trips they would take abroad together.

One of the most endearing incidents to Andrew and Ellen was their youngest daughter's concerns that Andrew would not get on the train in time with the luggage he had to shepherd. Everyone had a suitcase for the two-week journey plus their carry-on bags, and so, her worry was not frivolous at all, but of major concern. Disembarking from the train was a challenge. His daughter kept her eye on her father, slowing her progress off the car and everyone else's until she was assured "her Daddy" was safely esconced on the platform at the train station with all the bags accounted for. Of course, he had everything under full control, but it did take two cabs to transport the family and the luggage anywhere!

To add to the trial, Ellen succumbed to the allure of Murano glassware manufactured on an island just off Venice. This resulted in the appearance of yet another package to shepherd — a wooden carrier about the size of a brief case! Fortunately, the pieces arrived unbroken in Memphis and have been admired over the years, albeit mostly by his wife.

He did travel without his family, when it was not possible to include them. In 1978, in an attempt to warm the Cold War between the USSR and the U.S., a cultural and scientific exchange program had been agreed upon between the two countries. Dr. John Decker, Andrew's former Harvard Medical School Advisor, was in charge of constituting a U.S. Rheumatology Delegation to Russia. He included Andrew along with John Baum, Naomi Rothfield, Morris Ziff, and others.

They landed in Leningrad (St. Petersburg) to begin an experience that was to leave an indelible mark on the delegates about the tyranny and paranoia of the Communist state.

One of the delegates had been reading a book entitled "Russia and Its People" en route. Upon their disembarkation at customs, the book was confiscated and everyone was subsequently opened to thorough searches lasting a total of three hours for the entourage, presumably in search of similar "subversive propaganda" materials.

Living conditions were also trying and difficult in the USSR at that time. They had been alerted to the contamination of the water system with Giardia. Although the U.S. delegates had been warned to use bottled distilled water to drink and for brushing their teeth, Andrew was running low of his supply and elected to brush and rinse his mouth with tap water, reserving his bottle only for ingestion. However, even the water residue from rinsing contained sufficient numbers of Giardia to cause illness, as he discovered a few days later.

As it was, they had traveled by train from Leningrad to Moscow and were being received at an official banquet. At the banquet, the call of nature had come at the urging of Giardia, now multiplied in untold numbers. In such a public prominent building as the official banquet place, he could not imagine what he was to encounter. Coping without a toilet seat was bad enough, but there was no bathroom paper anywhere around. Not to be outdone, however, ingenuity surfaced. After utilizing all the scraps of paper in his wallet, he pulled out his handkerchief for the finishing touch and then gladly flushed it down into the Moscow drainage system hoping it would be removed before it reached the Volga.

Purchasing memorabilia of Russia for his family was another unique experience. The system of standing in long lines to select an item, followed by another lineup to make the payment, and finally in line again for the third time to retrieve the item was both aggravatingly time-consuming and awkward. Purchases were thereby necessarily limited. Whether this antiquated method of marketing was the result of insufficient availability of goods or the need to keep consumption rigidly controlled by the Communists was not clear to Andrew, or others in the entourage.

Each evening when he returned to his room, he found the contents of his suitcase displaced. Upon his return to Memphis, he found that two neat holes had been drilled on his suitcase, most likely to allow a probe to examine the contents before the plane had left Russia.

After the plane landed in London on its way to the U.S., all the delegates made it to the nearest Pub for a large serving of bitters. While Russia had a great culture in the past as exhibited by the opulence of the Czarist Palaces, the suffering of the masses must have been considerable to have resulted in the revolution, the delegates agreed among themselves at the Pub.

Andrew returned a "raging patriot," finding even the VA system a model of efficiency by comparison to operations in the USSR.

At this visit to Russia, he met a young scientist who expressed interest in visiting his laboratory in Memphis. Several years later, he did arrive for a three-week stay in Dr. Kang's laboratory.

At another international meeting where he traveled alone, he had been invited to chair a session at an International Meeting on Liver Cirrhosis in Muenster, Germany. The meeting organizer had trained earlier in Dr. Karl Piez's laboratory at the NIH.

A change in planes was made at Frankfurt. At Muenster, his luggage could not be found. After a quick trip to the nearest store for a few toiletries, he freshened up and went to the reception. Not knowing anyone, he sauntered towards a table where several oriental men sat together. He introduced himself when, suddenly, all three of the oriental men stood bolt upright and bowed.

One of them, Dr. Isao Okazaki, asked, "Are you the Professor Kang who published the collagenase paper with the diagram?"

"Why yes, I am."

"Oh my, I thought you would be a much older man."

And, another connection was made with this company of researchers from Keio University in Tokyo, Japan. Before the meeting was over, Dr. Kang was offered a verbal invitation to a meeting scheduled to be held in Japan within a year. This invitation was to open his way back to Asia and to initiate the training of many Postdoctoral Fellows from Japan in Dr. Kang's growing laboratory units with specialists in various biological sciences impacting on connective tissues and rheumatoid arthritis.

CHAPTER 14: RETURN TO ASIA AND BACK

In November of 1980, he took Ellen with him to Asia. Their older children were away in college and high school classes had already begun for their youngest. Ellen's technician, who knew Audrey well, stayed with her during their visit to Asia. Andrew had been invited to speak at a meeting in Kitakyushu, Japan after which they returned to Tokyo for interactions with various laboratory workers, including Dr. Yutaka Nagai who had spent time in Jerry Gross' laboratory.

This was their first visit to Japan and each was impressed with the economic strength of the country, the cleanliness of the cities, the diligence of her people, and the beauty of the countrysides.

Following these meetings, they flew to Seoul, Korea. This was his first return since his departure for the U.S. in 1955, twenty-five years earlier, and was Ellen's first visit to the land of her ancestors.

It was in November and the cold winds were already bearing down from Siberia, but their hearts were warmed by the visits with their many relations that lived within the Seoul area.

Each of Andrew's sisters scrutinized his wife closely wondering what it was about her that kept Tiger from returning back to Korea for nearly a quarter of a century.

Yes, she looked Korean, exhibited the social graces expected of a lady, but what kind of broken Korean was she speaking, they wondered? Somewhat disappointed that she could not speak their language like a Korean, they nevertheless communicated as best they could and things went pretty smoothly between Ellen and her sister-in-laws.

There was exchange of warmth and kindness between Andrew and his sisters allowing freer communication than there had been by correspondence or by telephone over the years since he had departed for college, years before. Somehow, he developed a sense that life had not gone well for two of his five siblings. In fact, he had an uncomfortable sense that he had perhaps failed to maintain his filial duties to his siblings, particularly to his younger brother, Pyo, who was not present. Correspondence had been poor between Pyo and himself, especially after Pyo's marriage a decade and a half before. Much earlier than that, with financial support from rental of their Father's property, Pyo had started college. Before long, he had to withdraw because of the intervention of an emotional illness. Although the illness had temporarily abated, he did not return back to college. Later, he married a pharmacist and in time the marriage produced two children. The first-born was a son followed by a daughter.

Seemingly, Pyo could not abide his son as he approached maturity, picking on him relentlessly, according to his wife. During a succeeding breakdown, he was institutionalized, to the relief of the wife. When he had gotten better again, she refused to have him returning home, electing to send him to a private sanatorium instead, which she forced herself to afford.

Hearing this, Andrew visited Pyo at the sanatorium with Ellen. Clearly, Pyo appeared sane, expressing a wish to join his family and evidencing normal behavior. Both Andrew and his wife were convinced of his readiness to return to his family.

After extensive negotiations with Pyo's wife, she agreed to have her husband to return home, provided arrangements would be made to have their son sent to America to study, in due course.

Andrew could not help but wonder if the stress of participating in the management of the family's life and finances together with their sisters after Andrew's departure for the U.S. might have contributed to Pyo's problems. On the other hand, he readily recalled his brother's quiet and withdrawn tendencies as a youngster and now could see that those very traits could have represented the expression of a disturbance in Pyo's perception of others and the world about him. Those were trying times and Pyo suffered equally, if not more, than he did through the horrors of the war and its aftermath because of his youth and immaturity.

He resolved to keep his end of the bargain with Pyo's wife and prayed that Pyo would maintain his sanity, going forward.

In addition to Pyo, his older sister, Ok Im, who's marriage he had brokered before he left for the U.S., was in clear need of financial help. In recent years, her husband exhibited the effects of chronic tuberculosis of the lungs and could only tolerate minimum employment with work brought to him at home. He was an educated man from a long line of scholars and so was sought by other learned people to do piecemeal literary work for them at home. However, there was not enough earned to educate their daughters and Ok Im had to help with finances by taking on menial tasks.

These facts had not been transmitted to Andrew by correspondence, but clarified themselves rather painfully during this visit, not only by observation but by input from each of Andrew's other sisters.

Fortunately, each of his three younger sisters had completed their college education and had married educated, healthy men who provided for their growing families quite well.

He was also startled to find he had lost command of his native language, forgetting many words! It was difficult to explain matters and things in Korean. He had an odd feeling that in some ways Korea, the language and social culture, had become somewhat foreign to him. He was saddened in a strange sort of way, recognizing that he had clearly become very American, no longer a pure Korean, as a natural outcome of transplanting to the other culture.

On the brighter side of this visit, Andrew could see that Korea was emerging as a free market society after the Park Chung Hee dictatorship. The effects of Park's tenure had brought the country out of the quagmire of an undisciplined, unregulated near anarchial state to a regimented, better disciplined nation of workers seeking to better themselves by hard work.

Andrew recalled reading with great dismay many years earlier that the economic cognoscenti of the day had predicted that South Korea was the least likely of the emerging nations of the world to recover economically. And, to his delight, he could clearly see that they were wrong, wrong, wrong! Instead, a sort of an economic miracle had occurred.

He departed hopeful that the corner had been turned and the fledgling democracy would survive, provided the Communists were held at bay.

Back in Memphis, he followed up on his resolve, arranging for Pyo's son to come to study at Wofford College in Spartanburg, S.C.—the same college that had offered him a scholarship to the U.S. and provided the environment and personnel who helped him make a smooth transition to this culture. He accompanied his brother's son, Paul, to Wofford

College and saw to his periodic visits with the rest of his family in Memphis.

Sometime following these developments, a near life-threatening experience occurred when the car he was driving, a Datsun, collided with a Volvo on a bridge spanning a busy, major interstate highway. It was evening and he was on his way home when this occurred. His car was totaled, squashed near the railing, but he was alive, though badly injured. Amazingly, he was not tossed over the bridge onto the busy highway below! The passenger in the steeled Volvo was merely jolted without any visible damage to either his car or to himself, attesting to the greater safety of the Volvo from either the passenger's or driver's point of view.

The injury he sustained resulted in hospitalization for about a week in neck traction. Fortunately, no bones had been fractured, but the trauma to the ligaments of his neck and upper back, previously affected by spondylitis reawakened pain and discomfort. Bracketed in a neck brace, he was able to resume activities but it took time to heal the traumatized ligaments. All the while, he revisited the pathophysiological changes occurring at the collagenous sites damaged during this accident.

Over time, Andrew had envisioned that his success in Memphis might open opportunities elsewhere. And indeed, only a few years after the automobile accident, he was being actively sought by a number of outside institutions.

He made three visits to the University of Iowa to possibly head their Rheumatology Division. After seriously considering various aspects of their offer, in the end, he did not accept the position because no significant advantage seemed apparent for the rest of his family.

Later, serious consideration was being made for a move to UCLA to head the Rheumatology Division there with the promise of an Endowed Chair to follow. However, the Chair was not yet free and real estate costs were found to be extremely exorbitant in California. Still, he was seriously considering the move and returned to UCLA on three occasions to evaluate the advantages of such a change.

At this time, he was visited by Dr. John Griffith, the Chairman of the Department of Pediatrics who was appointed as the Head of the Search Committee for a new Chairman of the Department of Medicine at the University of Tennessee itself following the departure of Dr. Gene Stollerman for Dartmouth, N.H. Dr. Griffith asked why he had not submitted his candidacy for the position and requested his Curriculum Vita (CV) be forwarded.

Without fully understanding what the Chairman's job would entail, he took up the challenge and followed through with the submission of his CV.

After due process, he was selected as the Chairman of the Department of Medicine at UT, Memphis in 1982. When Dean Robert Summitt offered him the Chairmanship, Andrew was ready to accept the challenge. He was almost as delighted as when he was offered the scholarship to Wofford College many years before.

With this appointment, Andrew became the first Asian to be appointed as Chairman of any Department of Internal Medicine in a U.S. based medical school. Fully aware of this, he was determined to do well by wisely expanding and improving his Department in the three areas over which medical school departments had a mission: teaching, patient care, and research.

CHAPTER 15: CHAIRMAN OF MEDICINE

In 1982, Andrew took up the challenge as Chairman of the Department of Internal Medicine at the University of Tennessee, a post he was to hold for ten years. Now, considerations had to be made for the good of the whole Department, not merely his own clinical and research areas of interest.

Some Divisions were without leadership so among the initial moves he made was to recruit Dr. John Hoidal from Minnesota to head the Pulmonary Division.

Another important area was to recruit a respected, nationally recognized individual to head the Cancer Center. For a number of years, Andrew's predecessor, Dr. Gene Stollerman, had searched for such a leader without success. Andrew had served with Dr. Alvin Mauer, then head of St. Jude Children's Research Hospital, at Dr. Stollerman's request, searching without success for such an individual. Upon Andrew's ascension to the Chair, Dr. Mauer became available for recruitment, stepping down as head of St. Jude Research Hospital. With Chancellor Jim Hunt's support, Dr. Mauer was successfully recruited to head the Cancer Center at the University of Tennessee.

Other recruitments followed, but each one became progressively more difficult because of dwindling State revenues and the Chancellor's administrative extension of recruiting preferences to other Departments, particularly in the Basic Sciences. While Andrew was in favor of raising the standard of the Basic Science Departments, he was increasingly disappointed that these were. made not in addition to the recruiting efforts in the College of Medicine, but rather in lieu of any recruitment they intended to make to shore up the clinical departments at the University.

Several difficult experiences also arose. One in particular where a painful decision had to be made against his personal feelings bothered him immensely. A former Boston neighbor of his had been recruited to head a Division in the Department of Medicine. Unwittingly, he had not abided by established University protocol. Maneuvering to allow grace to all parties concerned, he allowed the individual to depart for another position elsewhere, preserving his reputation and the University's established rules.

Several years into the Chairmanship, Andrew was named the Goodman Professor, an honor that he continues to hold.

Within the first 5 years of his Chairmanship, he had doubled the Department's research funding from the NIH.

Gradually however, the Chairman's job lost its sweet savor. The growth of Managed Medical Care was sucking the lifeblood out of medical schools everywhere. The administrative hassles of fighting to hold on to the dollars the Department of Medicine legitimately earned, keeping other Departments from wrenching dollars away by one ruse or another, were unbearable to him.

One of his Division heads, Dr. Bill Rosenberg, a mercurial intellectual, capsulized his growing sentiment in a nutshell when he asked, "How does it feel to be a mixed bag where for the first time you're working for everyone else, but not yourself?"

"With every decision, you make 9 enemies and 1 ingrate, just like Roosevelt said when asked about how it felt to be the President, right?" he asked.

Damage control became more important than improving the Department. For example, he had been working with the Regional Medical Center (RMC) Hospital Director and successfully got them to agree to compensate his Department of Medicine for patient care rendered into two separate coffers, one to UT and the other to the University of Tennessee Medical Group or UTMG.

Prior to this, the Department of Medicine was receiving $400,000 from the RMC for services rendered. Now, they would receive nearly 10 times this amount, by Andrew's accounting. This arrangement would allow persons to be recruited into the tenure track to be paid through UTMG. Monies in the UT coffer expired annually on June 30th. Since UTMG was a nonprofit Corporation, monies could be carried into the next year, rendering great flexibility in accommodating salaries as well as in the matter of recruitment of personnel.   .

Soon Andrew learned that the Dean's Administrator was claiming half of the monies for operations in other Departments. Argument with the Dean and his Administrator over this matter became an annual exercise in frustration. It soon became clear to him that at this rate the Department of Medicine could no longer grow, and that he was merely keeping the Department from deteriorating, if that.

In 1992, after a decade at the helm, he decided to step down. No amount of cajoling by the Dean to stay on as Chairman would make him change his mind.

About the same time, he was still being recruited to other Chairmanships, elsewhere. He considered each for a while, but concluded that while they were different venues, the bag of tricks available, while new, would in the long run be the same as he had dealt with in Memphis.

In addition, he was being invited to consider Deanships at two centers, the University of Hawaii and the University of South Alabama. After visits to each of these centers, he concluded that both would be like jumping into the fire from a hot, hot pan.

Therefore, he made a conscious decision to go back to what he knew how to do rather well. He was ready to return to and focus on research, no question about that.

CHAPTER 16: BACK TO FULL-
TIME RESEARCH

Back into research on a full-time basis, he realized that others in research no longer regarded him as a serious investigator, considering him to be merely an administrator. One of them in his own group had even suggested that he undertake a sabbatical to catch-up and gain credibility. But this was not to his interest at that time.

The RO1 grants he held ever since his move to Memphis had not been renewed and the recent review on his VA grant submission for continuation did not reach the fundable level, almost lending credibility to those who thought him out of step with the state of research in connective tissue diseases.

These reversals had occurred at a time when a funding nadir had coincided at the two major funding agencies for this type of research, the NIH and the VA systems

However, he still had a large source of research funding from an NIH Specialized Center of Research (SCOR) in Rheumatoid Arthritis, which was subsequently refunded in

1992 for another five years. And not long after his return to full-time research, both of his VA and Individual Research or R01 NIH funding requests were awarded, once again.

A gradual transformation had taken place in his approach to research over the years. Whereas he had looked at RA straight in the eye, so to speak, first looking for the enzyme involved in the destruction of collagen and then defining the structural features of the tissue that rendered it susceptible to destruction, now his attention was focused on the immunologically important factors that regulate the various steps involved in the inflammatory process underlying RA.

Once the collagen scaffold of the extracellular matrix composed of the interstitial collagens (types I, II and III) is acted upon by collagenase at a single site through the triple helical molecule, the fragments spontaneously denature at body temperatures. These collagen fragments, reproducibly formed through the action of specific enzymes, act to initiate specific immunological cellular responses after binding to various tissue and immunologically important cells.

Studies of cell-mediated immunity induced by collagen peptides had been championed earlier by members of his group including Postlethwaite, Stuart, and Townes. The immunological events resulting from immunization of rodents with type II collagen had also been characterized and compared to patients with RA (Stuart, Cremer, Townes, Hufstutter). And importantly, a peptide fragment initiating the immunological response had been identified (Seyer, Hasty, Terato, Cremer, Stuart, Townes).

Both chemotactic and inhibitory factors affecting cellular migration and function had been defined and the effect of interleukins and lymphokines on the regulation of collagen synthesis in cell systems, in wound healing and tissue repair had been reported earlier by Postlethwaite and others in his group.

Using an animal model of type II collagen-induced arthritis in rodents that was first described by Trentham, Townes, and himself, demonstration that the intravenous administration of native type II collagen could suppress antigen-specific arthritis in the rat was reported by Cremer, Hernandez, Townes, Stuart,and Kang. Accordingly, a series of logical studies to identify immunosuppressive epitope determinants that would confer protection against collagen-induced arthritis, or tolerance, became a major objective of his research.

A tolerogenic T-cell epitope of type II chick collagen that suppressed arthritis in a specific arthritis susceptible strain of mice had been identified within residues CII 245-270 with Myers, Stuart, Seyer and himself.

By introducing specific site-directed substitutions within the immunodominant T cell epitope, an analog peptide was developed which is capable of down regulating immune response and arthritis via immune deviation as reported with Myers, Miyahara, Terato, Seyer, Stuart, Rosloniec, Brand, Kawamura, Esaki, Gumanovskaya, and others. The mechanism by which these events occur at the cellular level have also been studied and partially defined.

Using the murine model, tolerogenic determinants of collagen have been identified using a peptide analog of type II collagen as reported with Myers, Tang, Rosloniec, Stuart, and Chiang. Cytokine responses to intravenous tolerization with type II collagen have been defined with Gumanovskaya, Myers, Rosloniec and Stuart. Interestingly, genetic ablation of cyclooxygenase-2 was shown to prevent the development of murine autoimmune arthritis with Myers, Postlethwaite, Rosloniec, Morham, Shlopov, Goorha, and Ballou.

Studies continue in these areas, with great anticipation that some of their innovative approaches in the laboratory might soon lead to the development of therapeutically successful means to reverse, alleviate, or even prevent the clinically devastating effects of connective tissue diseases.

Following up on studies of the mechanism underlying the interaction of platelets with collagen upon disruption of the endothelial surfaces of blood vessels, the platelet membrane receptor for A1(type 1), molecular size (M_r) of 65 kDa, was identified by molecular cloning techniques. Another platelet receptor for type III collagen, M_r 47 kDa, has also been found. The residues of importance for collagen interaction for each type-specific platelet receptor as well as the functional significance of both active peptides in combination and individually under flow conditions have also been studied with Chiang.

The studies completed and ongoing could easily lead to the development of peptide sequences that could counter the effects of the response of platelets to exposed collagen molecules upon denudation of the vascular endothelium.

Dr. Kang continues to direct the research for the area of his current interest while recruiting, encouraging, and overseeing the growth of his Connective Tissue Division. Researchers in related areas of interest, with either M.D. or Ph.D. degrees, or both, continue to be included to enlarge the scope of the group's endeavors. Scores of trainees at the pre and postdoctoral levels have come and gone. Selective ones are retained, such that the number of his group cannot be accommodated at one sitting at the Christmas gathering usually hosted at his home nearly every year.

He has a remarkable ability to accommodate researchers of various backgrounds, paving a way for each, bridging gaps, coping with financial inequities by reallocating resources obtained from somewhere, all the while fostering research, cajoling all to excellence, thereby ensuring stability and completion of work initiated while winning loyalty and altruism for his group.

He continues to serve on various campus, national and international committees having to do with biomedicine in general, research in specific areas, the conduct of clinical research, as considered by the Arthritis Foundation and the General Clinical Research Centers for the NIH, and on the boards of scientific journals.

In addition to the Russell L. Cecil Award that had been given by the Arthritis Foundation in 1971, he received the Philip Hench Award in 1977. The Founders Medal was received from the Southern Society for Clinical Investigation in 1994 and he was elected to the rank of Master by the American College of Rheumatology in 1999.

Andrew continued to oversee the wellbeing and education of his brother's son in the U.S. and gave support to his eldest sister, whose husband eventually passed away.

Similarly all the while, Andrew continued in like manner with his family, planning ahead, coping with challenges, ready to support his children through their educational goals, whatever they were without any financial constraints, and he also managed to include wonderful family vacations that would live forever in their memories.

Each summer, the family made a two-week trip to somewhere. It could be Cape Cod, New Hampshire, New York, Montreal, Washington, D.C., the Grand Canyon, San Francisco and Yosemite Valley, Disney Land, Spartanburg, South Carolina and Myrtle Beach, or Florida from Destin to St. Augustine and Cape Canavaral including numerous return visits to Sanibel and Captiva Islands. Even Europe was a treat on two occasions for the entire family. Korea and Japan were also visited with them by two of the three daughters. The eldest could not join them to visit Asia because of her internship schedule but was able to join them along with her husband and sons a few years later.

All three of his daughters elected to study medicine, two at Brown University and the middle one at the University of Pennsylvania. The eldest specialized in Dermatology, the middle in Radiology, and the youngest in Obstetrics and Gynecology in Maternal-Fetal Medicine.

Each married stellar young men of Caucasian origin, the eldest to a fellow medical student who became a Cardiologist, the middle daughter to a Brown classmate of hers who became a Computer Engineer, and the youngest to a Vanderbilt Internist who later won an MBA degree as well.

In time, Andrew saw the arrival of Grandchildren whose features blend Asian and Caucasian characteristics most beautifully. Their growth and development delight him immensely. Invariably, their visits are too short and too far between for him.

At the time of this writing, there are four of them, three Grandsons and one Granddaughter, with another on the way for his youngest daughter, a male by modern sonography. Each of those already born calls him "Hapu" because the word for grandfather in Korean, Harrabuji, is a bit too difficult for little ones to pronounce and the contraction Habu is likely to be converted to Hapu. So, Hapu it has been and will undoubtedly continue to be forever.

Over the span of 28 years, even their housekeeper has found him a friend and counselor. He has also been her personal financier for unexpected needs at no financial interest charges to her. As a black single mother on minimum wage, she had not been able to obtain credit at the local banks. After her initial timid approach to him, his heart was touched by her incredible disadvantage in our system leading him to support her in worthy financial stakes. Consequently with his wife's concurrence, he has helped in the down payment and repair of her home, payment against some of the debts incurred in the education of her children, as well as in the down payment for another house to augment her income as rental property. Repayment over the years, but never with added interest, has always been on time. She continues to this day to maintain their home with the assurance that should a legitimate financial need arise, she had a source of reliable help she could invariably depend on.

In the year 2001, Andrew's contributions in the study of rheumatoid arthritis and the biology and regulation of collagen under normal and pathological conditions were recognized by the Ho-Am Committee of his former homeland, Korea. Awards had been given annually through the aegis of SamSung Corporation for the previous 10 years in Medicine, Science, Engineering, the Arts, and in Human Services. These awards are the highest the country can give and are considered the Korean equivalent to the Nobel Awards. He was selected to receive the prestigious award in Medicine for the year 2001.

Interestingly, after receiving the Ho-Am award, when asked by one of his grandsons to divulged his roadmap to success, he listed three rules that guided and still guide him today: 1) Use your head, 2) Stick to it, and then 3) Work harder than the next fellow. Indeed, these have been the triad of mottos he has followed throughout his career.

To add further to the honors accrued in the year 2001, his group garnered two large SCOR awards from the NIH, one for Rheumatoid Arthritis and the other for Scleroderma. Director of the former was Dr. Kang himself and the Director of the latter was Dr. Arnold Postlethwaite, whom Dr. Kang had recruited years earlier. Dr. Kang also won an NIH Bonus Core Grant offering scientific core services and seed money to enhance the climate of research in connective tissue biology and pathology at the University of Tennessee.

Adding further to their solid financial status in research and training, the State of Tennessee awarded the group a million dollars each year for five years as a Center of Excellence in Connective Tissue Diseases. Thus armed, the group continues to work towards unraveling the mechanism of disease production and means to regulate it under the guidance of the man who traveled alone from Korea to the new land, America, so long ago.

The Laboratory Sciences Research and Development Division of the Office of Research and Development of the Veterans Health Administration awarded Dr. Kang the William S. Middleton Award for the year 2003 for outstanding achievement in biomedical research. It is the highest honor for scientific achievement given by this organization. Dr. Kang's "contributions to the understanding and treatment of connective tissue diseases, particularly rheumatoid arthritis, his exemplary record of involvement in, and service to the VA and to the biomedical profession" were duly recognized.

More recently, the lock to the dark cache mired deep in his mind has had to be opened to pry out the painful details of the scenes and feelings of that awful time in late September of 1950 in order to gather the facts for this writing. Even now, excavation of those past events is not without consequences. But they take the form of a deeper setting of the eyes, a dilation of the pupils, a pinching of the nostrils and a tightening of the lips, with perhaps, some gritting of the teeth, in between occasional sighs where exhalation is nearly twice as long as inhalation. The bad dreams with the undecipherable words shouted in fright and anger have gone.

While the where about of his Father had never been revealed or discovered, he has somehow accommodated this insoluble void, perhaps aided by the recognition that his Father's suffering must surely be over, now nearly fifty years later.

The cumulative effects of life's events since his encounter with Colonel Crumpton in Seoul have been a salve to the wounds incurred to his battered spirit more than fifty years ago. The kindnesses and considerations expressed to him in various ways by people in the United States soothed and helped in the healing process. Still a Tiger to the core, occasionally licking the last vestiges of the nearly healed scar, he sometimes wonders what life would have been like if his parents had survived the Communist invasion.

CHAPTER 17: CREDITS

Dr. Kang's contributions in biomedicine involve the study of collagen, its structure, biology, and regulation under normal and pathological conditions. Clearly, the beginning of his long and illustrious career to understand the nature of collagen stemmed from his own personal experience with rheumatoid arthritis following his first year in medical school. But, neither these events nor his accomplishments could have come about were it not for the people who touched his life in such a way as to ensure the direction that his walk through life would take.

Many of these special individuals have been mentioned in this work. Several bear repeating because of the special importance of their contributions to his life. Beside his immediate family, as one who shared his life for over four decades, I would include his Aunt who was by his side when he found his Mother; his Uncle Choi Han Woong who was always there; Chung Byung Uk and his family who provided warmth and housing in his bid to complete high school after he was orphaned; Colonel Sidney Crumpton who selected him for the scholarship that brought him to America; Frank Logan and his wife who practically adopted him into their family at Wofford College; Dr. and Mrs. Johnson, several of his special Harvard classmates, Dr. John Decker, Dr. Ellis Dresner, Dr. Karl Piez, Dr. Jerry Gross, Dr. Gene Stollerman, Dr. Robert L. Summitt, and every one of the investigators who worked with him in his journey through the hills and valleys of research.

At the University of Tennessee, his collaborators included Ed Beachey (Infectious Disease), Kenzo Hashimoto and Tamotsu Kanzaki (Dermatology), Bill Duckworth (Endocrinology), John Whitaker (Neurology), Charles Arkin (practice of Rheumatology), Izak Ofek (Visiting Scientist from Tel Aviv, Israel), Gene Stollerman (Chairman, Dept. of Medicine), Alex Townes (Rheumatology), Stan Kaplan (Rheumatology), Larry Cagen (Pharmacology), Jim Pitcock (Pathology), T.J. Yoo (Allergy/Immunology), John Hoidal (Pulmonary), Gary Olson (Veterinary Services), John Fain (Biochemistry), A. Rinaldy (Immunology), Grant Sommes (Statistics), and several others.

Recruitees and Postdoctoral Fellows who contributed to the unraveling of connective tissue biology and pathology in Andrew's and his coworkers' laboratories included D. Katzman, J. Seyer, A. Postlethwaite, S. Dixit, C. Mainardi, J. Stuart, T. Chiang, M. Cremer, K. Hasty, G. Smith, M. Hibbs, L.K. Myers, D. Trentham, A. Hernandez, R. Raghow, K. Terato, R. Gupta, K. Kashiwazaki, R. Aycock, G. Stricklin, M. Ochs, J. Keiski-Oja, H. Poppleton, W. Watson, R. Endres, J. Armendari-Borunda, R. Reife, K. Ohyama, L. Ballou, C. Simkevich, D. Spinella, K. Katayama, E. Rosloniec, D. Brand, X. Ye, N. Roy, H. Miyahara, S. Kawamura, Y. Esaki, M. Gumanovskaya, J. Aelion, B. Tang, K. McKown, L. Carbonne, K. Lohr, and several others.

Throughout Dr. Kang's career, he has been involved with the training of investigators at many levels (graduate and postdoctoral students, visiting scientists) from many parts of the world. It is remarkable that after the return of students to their mother country, another is sent for training. Thus, he has attained international status as a leader and teacher of caliber and personal grace.

With regard to one of these countries, the one that gave him life and launched him toward the west, Korea, he was responsible for training the first group of rheumatologists in Internal Medicine. Each of these rheumatologists returned to Korea and now heads the major rheumatology units of medical schools: Dr. Ho Youn Kim, former Chief of Rheumatology at Catholic Medical Center now Chairman of the Department of Internal Medicine, who is also Secretary/Treasurer of the Korean Rheumatism Association; Dr. Seong Yong Kim, Chief of Rheumatology at Hanyang Medical School; and, Dr. Yun Woo Lee, Chief of Rheumatology at Baik Hospital, Inje Medical School. Dr. Kang is regarded as the Father of the Rheumatology Movement in Internal Medicine in Korea.

In addition, credits are due to individuals and groups who in acknowledgement of his research accomplishments and leadership had invited him as a speaker or guest faculty across this nation as well as internationally.

Several of these invitations opened his vision to new possibilities, in particular, when he served as the Chairman of a Scientific Workshop on "The Biology and Pathology of Acquired Connective Tissue Diseases" for the National Institute of Arthritis Musculoskeletal and Skin Diseases and the National Arthritis Advisory Board in 1991.

Internationally, hosts in the following countries and cities where he had been invited to speak or to be part of symposia deserve acknowledgement for bringing cultural interests into his life [England (London, Cambridge), France (Paris),

Germany (Munich), Portugal (Oporto), Russia (Moscow), Turkey (Ankara), China (Beijing), Japan (Mishima, Kyoto, Tokyo), Korea (Seoul, Kyongju, Cheju), and Indonesia (Bali)].

Needless to say, he will continue to foster the advance of scientific knowledge for a few additional years to come, but when the time to relinquish leadership of his cadre of excellent investigators arrives, he would know, like a Tiger, true to form.

Printed in the United States
47776LVS00002B/109-111

9 781424 110179